The Complete Taping Handbook

of related interest

Osteopathic and Chiropractic Techniques for the Foot and Ankle
Clinical Understanding and Advanced Treatment Applications
and Rehabilitation for Manual Therapists
Giles Gyer and Jimmy Michael with Dr Kumar Kunasingam
ISBN 978 1 83997 201 0
eISBN 978 1 83997 202 7

Fascia in Sport and Movement, Second Edition
Robert Schleip, Jan Wilke and Amanda Baker
Foreword by Thomas W Findley
ISBN 978 1 91208 577 4
eISBN 978 1 91208 578 1

Fascial Stretch Therapy, Second Edition
Ann Frederick and Chris Frederick
Forewords by Thomas W Myers and Benny F Vaughn
ISBN 978 1 91208 567 5
eISBN 978 1 91208 568 2

Hip and Knee Pain Disorders
An Evidence-Informed and Clinical-Based Approach
Integrating Manual Therapy and Exercise
Edited by Benoy Mathew, Carol Courtney and Cesar Fernandez-de-las-Penas
Forewords by Alison Grimaldi, Vikas Khanduja and Cara L Lewis
ISBN 978 1 91342 613 2
eISBN 978 1 91342 614 9

Spine and Joint Articulation for Manual Therapists
Giles Gyer, Jimmy Michael and Ben Calvert-Painter
ISBN 978 1 90914 131 5
eISBN 978 1 91208 518 7

Advanced Osteopathic and Chiropractic Techniques for Manual Therapists
Adaptive Clinical Skills for Peripheral and Extremity Manipulation
Giles Gyer and Jimmy Michael
ISBN 978 0 85701 394 1
eISBN 978 0 85701 395 8

THE COMPLETE TAPING HANDBOOK

Biomechanical, Sports Rigid Taping
and K-Taping for Manual Therapists

Ben Calvert-Painter and Tim Allardyce

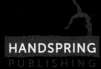

HANDSPRING
PUBLISHING

First published in Great Britain in 2025 by Handspring
Publishing, an imprint of Jessica Kingsley Publishers
Part of John Murray Press

1

A CIP catalogue record for this title is available from the
British Library and the Library of Congress

ISBN 978 1 80501 273 3
eISBN 978 1 80501 274 0

Printed and bound in China by Leo Paper Products Ltd

Jessica Kingsley Publishers' policy is to use papers that are natural, renewable
and recyclable products and made from wood grown in sustainable
forests. The logging and manufacturing processes are expected to conform
to the environmental regulations of the country of origin.

Handspring Publishing
Carmelite House
50 Victoria Embankment
London EC4Y 0DZ

www.handspringpublishing.com

John Murray Press
Part of Hodder & Stoughton Limited
An Hachette UK Company

Contents

Preface II

Acknowledgements 13

Glossary 15

I. **Introduction** 21
    What are the best brands and tapes?   22
    A brief history of taping   26
        Rigid tape   26
        K-tape/kinesio tape   28
        Biomechanical tape   31
    Questions to address before using tape   33
        Important tips   36
    Contraindications and considerations for taping   36
    Pre-tape preparation   37
    Overview of application   39
    Complications from poor taping technique   40
    Aftercare   41
        Tape removal   42
    References   43

2. **Lumbar Spine** 47
    Research evidence   47
    Techniques   49

Rigid taping of the lumbar spine   49

K-taping of the lumbar spine: standard technique   51

K-taping of the lumbar spine: pyramid technique   53

Biomechanical taping of the lumbar spine: arrow technique   56

Biomechanical taping of the lumbar spine: cross taping technique   57

References   59

3. Thoracic Spine and Ribs 61

Research evidence   61

Techniques   62

K-taping for the thoracic spine: rib pain   62

K-taping for the thoracic spine: trapezius and rhomboid pain   64

K-taping for the thoracic spine: mid thoracic pain   65

Biomechanical taping for the thoracic spine: postural support   67

References   68

4. Shoulder 71

Research evidence   71

Techniques   73

Rigid taping of the shoulder: shoulder support   73

K-taping of the shoulder: rotator cuff   75

K-taping of the shoulder: acromioclavicular joint   77

K-taping of the shoulder: biceps   78

Biomechanical taping of the shoulder: internal rotation (cocking phase)   79

Biomechanical taping of the shoulder: external rotation (throwing phase)   81

Biomechanical taping of the shoulder: biceps/supraspinatus   82

References   84

5. Elbow 87

Research evidence   87

Techniques   88

Rigid taping of the elbow   88

K-taping of the elbow: lateral epicondylitis   91

K-taping of the elbow: medial epicondylitis   92

Biomechanical taping of the elbow: deloading lateral epicondylitis   93

Biomechanical taping of the elbow: deloading medial epicondylitis   95

References   97

6. **Wrist and Hand** 99

Research evidence   99

Techniques   100

Rigid taping for thumb support   100

K-taping for carpal tunnel syndrome   102

Biomechanical taping for carpal tunnel syndrome   103

Biomechanical taping for De Quervain's tenosynovitis   104

References   106

7. **Hip** 107

Research evidence   107

Techniques   108

K-taping of piriformis   108

Biomechanical taping for trochanteric bursitis   110

Biomechanical taping for deloading iliopsoas   112

References   113

8. **Knee** 115

Research evidence   115

Techniques   117

Rigid taping of the medial and lateral knee   117

K-taping for retro-patellar inflammation/maltracking patella   119

K-taping of the knee for hamstring strain   121

Biomechanical taping for deloading quadriceps/maltracking patella   122

Biomechanical taping for lateral collateral sprains/meniscal support 123

Biomechanical taping for medial collateral sprains/medial meniscus tear 125

Biomechanical taping for deloading hamstrings 126

Biomechanical taping for deloading tibialis anterior (shin splints). 127

References 129

9. **Ankle** 133

Research evidence 133

Techniques 135

Rigid taping for ankle support 135

K-taping for ankle sprains 138

K-taping for Achilles tendonitis 139

Biomechanical taping for deloading the Achilles tendon 140

Biomechanical taping for inversion support 141

Biomechanical taping for eversion support/flat feet 143

References 144

10. **Foot** 147

Research evidence 147

Techniques 148

Rigid taping for turf toe 148

Rigid taping for plantar fasciitis 150

Biomechanical/k-taping for hallux valgus 152

Biomechanical taping for plantar fasciitis: toe wrap 154

Biomechanical taping for plantar fasciitis: sling 156

References 157

11. **Lymphatic Taping** 159

Research evidence 159

Technique 161

K-taping for lymphatic drainage 161

References 162

12. Pregnancy 165

Research evidence   165

Techniques   166

   Biomechanical/k-taping for abdominal support: 1   166

   Biomechanical/k-taping for abdominal support: 2   168

References   169

Preface

My interest in the application and use of taping to help prevent injury is informed by experiencing multiple ankle injuries when I was younger and my involvement in different sports, including American football. After qualifying as an osteopath, I learned more about how tape can help in recovery and rehabilitation.

This book is aimed at giving the reader a broad perspective in the application of strapping and taping within the clinic and at the pitch-side. Although it does not describe every single type of application and injury (the book would be huge!), the hope is that it covers everything you need to understand how to tape, the different types of tape that can be used, and the rationale for using each one. Once you have this understanding, you can choose the appropriate tape for any indication and apply it accordingly – whether you need to support or restrict movement, or aid recovery.

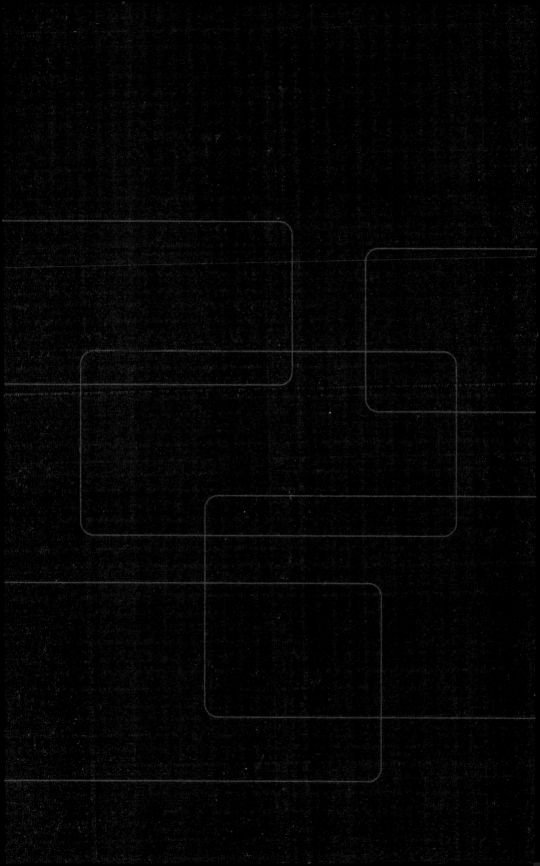

Acknowledgements

I would like to thank our model for her patience and resilience for the photoshoot, as it wasn't easy being taped so much! Thank you to my wife for tolerating my multiple late nights researching and writing, and for being the model in the pregnancy section. Thank you to Strapit for their permission in the use of their products.

Thank you to Tim for putting up with me and for all his contributions to the book including the design, production and overseeing all of the photos for this book.

And an obviously a huge thank you to our publishers for their patience and understanding during the production of this book.

Ben Calvert-Painter

Glossary

Abduction
A motion of a limb or appendage away from the midline of the body, or returning from an adducted position.

Acute
Conditions that are sudden or severe in recent onset (0–14 days).

Adduction
A motion of a limb or appendage towards the midline of the body, or returning from an abducted position.

Anatomical position
The body in an upright position, facing directly forward, feet flat and directed forward. The upper limbs are at the body's sides with the palms facing forward.

Anterior
Refers to the 'front', or lies in front.

Articulation
A location where two or more bones meet.

Bursa
A fluid-filled sac that lies near bony prominences and joints. The bursa

acts as a cushion and allows glide between structures such as muscles, ligaments and bones, thus reducing friction between these structures.

Bursitis
Inflammation of a bursa.

Caudal
Towards the tail or away from the head-end of the body.

Cephalad
Towards the head (or anterior extremity), a direction that in humans corresponds to superior.

Chronic
Conditions that are long lasting or that persist for more than three months.

Cranial
Of or relating to the bones of the head that cover the brain, or a direction towards the head.

Deep
Away from the surface or further into the body. As opposed to superficial.

Distal
A part of the body that is farther away from the centre of the body than another part.

Dorsal
Back portion of the body.

Dorsiflexion
Backward bending and contracting of your hand or foot. Can also be called extension of your foot at the ankle and your hand at the wrist.

Epicondyle
A rounded protuberance at the end of a bone, serving as a place of attachment for ligaments, tendons and muscles.

Eversion
Movement of the sole of the foot away from the median plane so that it faces a lateral direction.

Extension
A movement that increases the angle between two body parts.

Fascia
Layers of sheets of connective tissue that are below the skin. These tissues help to attach, stabilize, impart strength, maintain vessel patency, separate muscles and enclose different organs.

Flexion
A movement that decreases the angle between two body parts.

Greater trochanter
A large protrusion located at the proximal (near) and lateral (outside) part of the shaft of the femur (thigh bone).

Inferior
Towards the bottom or away from the head-end of the body.

Inversion
Movement of the sole of the foot inward towards the median plane so that it faces a medial direction.

Laminate
Placing one length of tape over another.

Ligament
A broad connective tissue connecting bone to bone.

Medial
Towards the middle or centre of the body.

Palmar
The palm or the anterior surface of the hand.

Palmar flexion
Movement of the hand and/or fingers towards the front of the forearm and/or hand (palm).

Plantar
Sole of the foot.

Plantar flexion
The extension of the ankle so that the foot points down and away from the leg, towards the floor.

Posterior
Refers to the 'back', or lies behind.

Pronation
Rotation of the forearm and hand so that the palm faces backwards or downwards, or a movement of the foot and leg in which the foot rolls inward with a depressed arch.

Prone
The body lying in a face down position.

Superficial
Closer to the surface of the body.

Superior
Towards the head-end of the body.

Supination
Rotation of the forearm and hand so that the palm faces forwards or upwards, or a movement of the foot and leg in which the foot rolls outwards with an elevated arch.

Tendon
A broad connective tissue connecting bone to muscle.

Tubercle
A small, rounded point of a bone.

Tuberosity
A moderate prominence where muscles and connective tissues attach.

CHAPTER 1

Introduction

Taping has been a part of physical therapy for decades. Initially, the only type of tape available was rigid sports tape or variations of this, such as zinc oxide tape. This type of taping is very effective in restricting movement and stabilising an area or joint, and so is used mainly in sports or situations where you want to either decrease the range of movement available in the joint, and/or prevent excessive movement in the area. Over the years we have also seen the development of kinesio tape or k-tape, and more recently biomechanical taping.

When someone is working or exercising, they can place excessive loading through contractile or non-contractile tissues, which can be sustained over long periods, i.e., posture or explosive movements during exercising or sports. This loading can also be due to abnormal directions of movement or a change in direction or biomechanical dysfunction, and over-loading or over-extension of movement. Also, excessive loading can come from fatigue, both mental and physical, repetition (repetitive strain injury), and can happen in both healthy or dysfunctional or injured tissue. Taping can help by protecting end range of movement of a joint(s) or muscle, by adding proprioception, improving fluid dynamics to an area, by taking some load or force from the tissues or by guiding the movement.

This book gives a brief history of some of the different types of taping available, the differences between them from their structure, to function and then application, and the rationale behind this. The

1

following chapters discuss research evidence for the taping of different areas and associated common injuries, and techniques are then described for rigid sports tape, k-tape and biomechanical tape, with the benefits given for each one. The reason for this is that we can use tape for different functions and rationales, be it from injury prevention, injury management, rehabilitation, postural and movement support, at different stages of healing, and to complement your current skills and treatments. The last part is key: taping should not override your treatment and supervision of your patients or clients – it is an additional therapy which can be used to enhance patient and client response to your skills (Montalvo et al., 2014).

What are the best brands and tapes?

The three different tapes also come in different sizes (as discussed in the individual technique sections of the book), but a brief overview is given below.

The range of brand names and products for rigid sports tapes and k-tape is huge, and from experience, some brands do not have consistent adhesive. We can highly recommend Strapit and Gripit tapes, by Strapit Medical and Sports Supplies, Australia. For biomechanical taping, at the time of writing, there are two brands: Dynamic Tape by Dymanic Tape Global and Active Tape by Gripit. Both are very good tapes, but for the purpose of this book we have used Active Tape by Gripit.

Rigid tape is commonly available in three widths: 25 mm, 38 mm and 50 mm. When using rigid tape, sometimes a sponge-type wrap is applied first as an underwrap (see Image 1.1).

K-tape normally comes in two widths of 50mm and 100mm, see Image 1.2 (we discuss what the different colours mean in the k-tape section that follows).

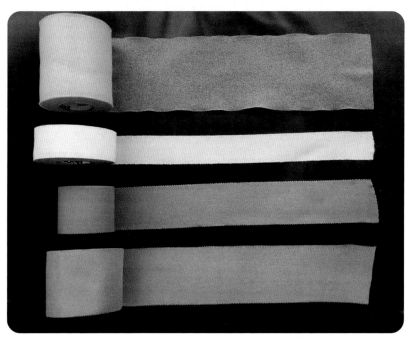

IMAGE 1.1 RIGID TAPE OF DIFFERENT WIDTHS, PLUS UNDERWRAP (TOP)

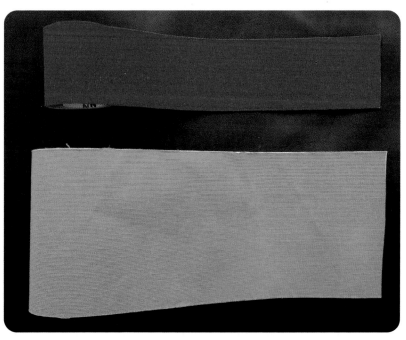

IMAGE 1.2 K-TAPE

K-tape can also be cut into different designs to help aid some of the techniques discussed in this book. Image 1.3 shows four different types of cuts.

Active Gripit biomechanical tape comes in three widths of 50 mm, 75 mm and 100 mm (see Image 1.4). These can also be cut straight or into a Y- or trouser cut (see Image 1.3).

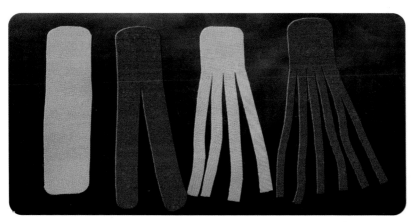

IMAGE 1.3 K-TAPE CUTS. FROM LEFT: STRAIGHT, Y-CUT (OR TROUSER CUT), AND TWO DIFFERENT FAN CUTS

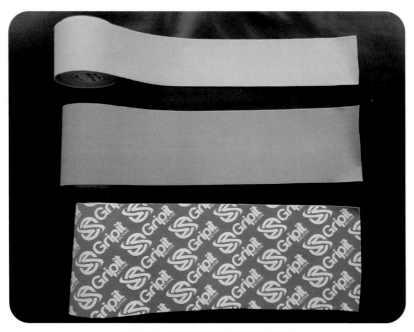

IMAGE 1.4 BIOMECHANICAL TAPE

Throughout the book we refer to laminating the biomechanical tape: this is basically layering a strip of biomechanical tape over another piece (see Image 1.5). This increases the elastic resistance of the layers of tape, and thus when there is an increased load, we can increase the strength of the tape recoil.

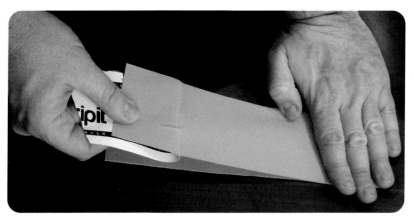

IMAGE 1.5 LAMINATING BIOMECHANICAL TAPE

Always invest in a good pair of tape scissors for cutting tape – not only do they cut the tape better than standard scissors, but they can cut tape faster when you have time restrictions either in clinic or pitch-side.

Image 1.6 shows two types of scissors: the first (left) is a standard taping scissor, and the second (middle) are 'Tuff cut' scissors. Tuff cut scissors have an angled design to the lower edge, which allows the scissors to be pressed against the skin without fear of cutting the skin. This is particularly useful when cutting dressings or rigid tape when underwrap is used.

On the right of the image is a 'tape shark'. Again, these are useful when taking off strapping with underwrap. These have a small blade and a rounded lower lip that can be pushed against the skin under tape when underwrap and bandages are used.

Tip: When using tape cutters or scissors, it is advisable to lubricate the tips with petroleum jelly and slide parallel to the skin.

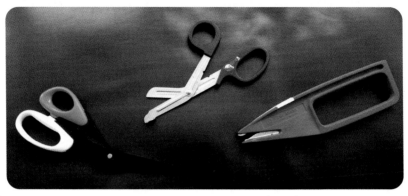

IMAGE 1.6 STANDARD TAPING SCISSORS (LEFT), TUFF CUT
SCISSORS (MIDDLE) AND A TAPE SHARK (RIGHT)

A brief history of taping

Rigid tape

The history of rigid taping is a little vague. The first use of an adhesive support to help stabilize joints is suggested by texts from ancient Roman and Egyptian times, which discuss the use of sticky cloths around limbs to help support and stabilize joints and muscles. Some say that the first type of surgical tape appeared in 1845, when Dr Horace Day and Dr William Shecut used a rubber adhesive applied to fabric strips, this being the predecessor for plasters, and Band Aid developed by Johnson and Johnson.

In 1885, Edward Cotterell, a surgeon at the University College Hospital, London, published a paper on the use of an adhesive strapping plaster (tape) titled: 'On some common injuries to limbs; Their treatment and after-treatment, including bone setting (so called) (Cotterell, 1885). In it, he discusses the application of adhesive strapping to 'rupture of the plantaris tendon', 'lawn tennis leg' and 'sprains of the ankle', and that the use of the tape provided support to joints and tissues, reduced pain and facilitated early ambulation.

Dr Virgil Gibney was inspired by Cotterell's work and found significant and immediate results in the use of tape, publishing *The Modern Treatment of the Sprained Ankle* in 1893 (Gibney, 1893). In 1895, he developed the 'Gibney Basketweave' method, which is still used and adapted today. He wrote about one particular episode where he had helped a bride walk down the aisle in a matter of just a few hours following an ankle sprain. This was revolutionary at the time, as people who had suffered a similar injury would take months to fully recover.

In 1899 Johnson and Johnson introduced their latest tape, a zinc oxide-based adhesive plaster, and thus rigid sporting tape came into being. Over the years this has been redeveloped and redesigned by many people into plasters, surgical tapes and strapping tapes, etc.

> During the first ever filmed American football game between Princeton and Yale in 1903, you can see players using athletic tape in an attempt to support joints and prevent injuries.

In the early stages of strapping, and most of the time within this book, rigid sports tape is applied directly onto the skin. This helps with the adhesion and support of movement, but can irritate the skin and make removing the tape painful. Therefore, in the 1970s underwrap was developed; this sponge-like material helps cushion the rigid support of the tape and reduces skin irritation, whilst making tape removal easier.

The main aim of rigid taping is to restrict movement and stabilize an area. The obvious disadvantage of this, therefore, is that joints or muscles potentially will not work efficiently or to their maximum because of the restriction of movement. But by limiting movement or supporting the end range of a joint, we are attempting to protect the joint, muscle or tissues. This is supported by research such as that by Gatt et al. (2023) and Clifford et al. (2020), and rigid taping is a recommended procedure in the benefit of athletic performance and injury prevention (Singh, 2019).

Benefits of rigid tape
- injury prevention
- muscle de-activation
- surrounding muscle support
- pain relief
- joint support and stability
- helps continued activity.

K-tape/kinesio tape

K-tape or kinesio tape (KT) was invented in the 1970s by Japanese chiropractor Kenzo Kase, but only gained worldwide recognition after its use in the 1988 Seoul Summer Olympics, when more and more therapists started to use it. Today, it is a very common sight to see colourful tapes on professional athletes and sportspeople, be it on their arms, legs or bodies. According to Kase (1994) it can promote several different therapeutic processes, including pain inhibition, improvement of circulation, lymphatic drainage and delaying of muscle soreness.

THE THEORY

The theory behind k-tape is that lifting the skin and soft tissue creates more space, thus decreasing pressure on capillaries and lymphatics that cross over fascia, which in turn increases the rate of healing and tissue repair (Skirven et al., 2011). By studying the effects of wrinkles in rabbits, Shim et al. (2003) found that the wrinkles compressed the skin but also elevated the space between the skin and fascia, which caused observable pressure variations and changes in fluid dynamics.

In addition, researchers have reported a range of benefits of using k-tape, including a beneficial effect on blood pressure and decrease in cardiac vagal tone at rest (Shah et al., 2018), a significant increase in circulation after total knee replacement surgery compared to controls (Windisch et al., 2017) and reduced analgesic consumption in patients following thyroidectomy (Genc et al., 2019). Studies by Cimino et al. (2018) and Slomka (2018) also found that k-taping caused changes to the skin and temperature respectively. Under laboratory investigation, Tu et al. (2016) found that k-tape 'reduced subcutaneous inter-tissue movement and paracutaneous translation in the superficial thoracolumbar fascia during lumbar flexion'. This is illustrated in Images 1.7a and 1.7b, the illustrations show the theory in how the recoil of the k-tape lifts the skin and fascia, thus creating more space and thus less pressure, therefore allowing improved movement of blood and lymphatic drainage.

Maggi et al. (2022) found a significant reduction in pain and functional improvement in patients with non-specific mechanical low back pain with the use of k-tape, and a systematic review by Artioli and Bertolini (2014) found that k-tape gave pain relief for between 24 hours to a week. For some patients, temporary relief from pain can make a huge difference, however, taping is not a stand-alone treatment, and is used as an adjunct to other therapies. In a systematic review by Tran et al. (2023), they found that k-tape provided improvement in both reducing pain and disability when applied to any region of the body. This was observed in the first five days of application, and improvement was also noted at four to six weeks of application. This supports the idea of using k-tape as an adjuvant to other treatments for musculoskeletal disorders.

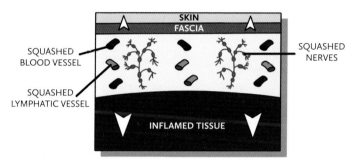

IMAGE 1.7A SHOWING COMPRESSED BLOOD AND LYMPHATIC VESSELS

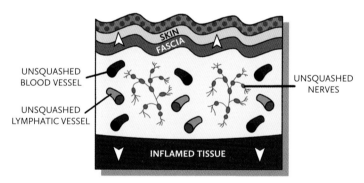

IMAGE 1.7B SHOWING THE THEORY OF HOW K-TAPE CREATES A LIFT AND RELEASE OF PRESSURE AROUND THE BLOOD AND LYMPHATIC VESSELS

Kase (2003) also suggested that k-tape can modulate muscle tone, and many studies have investigated whether k-tape can increase muscle strength and/or performance in healthy athletes (Mine et al., 2018; Csapo and Alegre, 2015; de Almeida Lins et al., 2013). The majority of studies have found that k-tape does not increase muscle strength, although some studies will report the opposite (Cochrane et al., 2023).

1

The main issue with these studies is that they are investigating how k-tape influences strength and performance in healthy athletes and tissues. This is like looking at how beneficial a stair lift is in a bungalow!

If the fluid dynamics of a tissue are not affected, applying a technique to help improve fluid dynamics is not going to make a difference; therefore a statistically significant change in muscle function in a healthy muscle will not be observed when taping. A meta-analysis by Yam et al. (2019) found an improvement in strength, but this was in people with muscle fatigue and chronic musculoskeletal diseases. This finding could have been as a result of improving the fluid dynamics of chronically compromised tissues, thus improving the performance of the muscles.

Kase (2003) repeatedly discusses the effect and benefit of k-tape in improving circulation and lymphatic drainage. In healthy tissue this is not statistically evident, but even so, in the field of elite sports where every athlete is seeking that 1% advantage over their competitors, it may give a physical or even mental edge to the healthy individual.

A study by Bérdi et al. (2015) examined 79 elite athletes and their thoughts towards placebo-induced performance enhancement. Over 80% thought that placebos could affect their performances positively, and just under half said they had experienced placebo effects in the past. 'When an athlete believes that an intervention is effective, the intervention will often result in a beneficial outcome, regardless of its merit' (Nichols et al., 2019).

This leads us on to the different colours of k-tape, and the question of what they all mean. The truth is, absolutely nothing, but studies have shown that the more colourful the tape, the better the placebo response. The other idea is that the various colours have different heat absorption properties, meaning that if an injury is chronic, using warm colours like red or pink will promote circulation and fluid dynamics, and if acute, using cool colours such as blue will be more soothing. However, there is no research evidence for this, only anecdotes and case studies.

In summary, the majority of evidence supporting k-tape comes not from the sports and athletics fields where it is mainly used, but from health care applications such as after injury or surgery (Chan et al., 2017; Hörmann et al., 2020), or for chronic tissue changes (Upadhaya et al., n.d.; Luo and Li, 2021).

Biomechanical tape

The rationale behind biomechanical taping is to 'deload' or take some load off tissues, i.e., joint capsule, ligaments, muscle or fascia. Before the advent of biomechanical tape, this deloading was achieved by using Theraband that would be strategically taped down, which was awkward and not always practical. In 2010, physiotherapists Ryan Kendrick and Ylva Kendrick developed Dynamic Tape, which imitated the action of Theraband, but could be applied in the desired position and was easier to use. As with k-tape and rigid tape, there have been different interpretations of this, and Active Tape by Strapit was developed for deloading tissues.

THE THEORY

McNeill and Pedersen (2016), Cook and Purdham (2009) and Soslowsky et al. (2002) describe conditions such as tendinopathy as the inability to dissipate or adapt to loading adequately, which can then result in maladaptive compensation in movement and behaviour. This then leads to the proposed three-stage process of tendon pathology: reactive tendinopathy, tendon disrepair (failed healing) and degenerative tendinopathy. The initial theory developed by Ryan Kendrick was that tape could be used to deload this area, and by removing some of the force and load, allow better movement and thus aid recovery.

BIOMECHANICAL TAPING PRINCIPLES

The three main principles in the application of biomechanical tape are:

- the tape must be applied over one or more joints
- it must be applied with the joint(s) in a shortened position
- the tape must have good anchors, as this helps with the biomechanical loading and function of the tape, and also in the prevention of traction blisters on the skin.

Biomechanical tape is applied differently to k-tape: where k-tape is commonly applied to an area in a lengthened position to help lift the skin, biomechanical tape is applied with the joint(s) in a shortened position, therefore giving more importance to the application, rather than placing stretch on the tape. This helps with the deloading or load absorption from the tissues and joints. The tape can either be applied in layers with degrees of overlay, or you can laminate the tape (as shown in Image 1.5). Laminating the tape increases its tension and load distribution qualities. By doing this, as the joint or muscle is extended, the elastic loading of the tape will increase, and when the muscle is contracted, the load on the muscle will be lightened or decreased during the movement. This can also help in guiding and even modifying movement.

A study by Song et al. (2022) found that biomechanical taping had a positive effect on endurance and muscular fatigue on plantar flexors in healthy adults. In the setting of plantar fasciitis, Kim and Lee (2023) found that biomechanical taping helped deload the plantar fascia, leading to improved biomechanics, reduced pain and enhanced healing of tissues. There are many other studies that support the theory of deloading the muscles to promote endurance, from the upper limb (Huang and Kim, 2020) to the lower back (Alahmari et al., 2020) to give but two examples.

In summary, each tape has its own properties, from how it is constructed and the theories behind its therapeutic effects, to its application and functions (see Table 1.1). Most importantly, do not forget that taping is rarely a treatment that is applied on its own – rather it is used to complement your skills, and can be added at different stages of recovery and rehabilitation.

Table 1.1 Summary of tape functions

	Rigid sports tape	Kinesiology tape	Biomechanical tape
Material	Cotton fabric	Cotton and Lycra	Nylon/Lycra and cotton
Percentage stretch	Nil	140–180%	200–250%
Rigid end point	Yes	Yes	No

Resistance and recoil	Nil	Weak	Strong
Direction of stretch	Nil	Longitudinal (2-way)	Longitudinal and transverse (4-way)
Position of application	Neutral / corrected/ shortened	Lengthened	Shortened
How it works	Mechanically restrictive	Works on the skin as an organ – influencing pain, blood and lymphatic flow and skin proprioception	Works to deload moving parts and protect tendons/ muscles/joints

Questions to address before using tape

- **Is the injury acute or chronic?**
  The reason we need to ask this is due to fluid dynamics. An acute injury triggers the body's inflammatory response, therefore applying a tight, non-stretching tape such as rigid tape, will constrict the movement of fluid in and out of injured tissues, which compromises the natural healing processes and is also painful for the patient. Hence when an injury is in the acute phase, we may need to give support which is not too restrictive and will allow for swelling to take place. We can also help with inflammation by creating an environment to ease fluid movements and drainage (see more on this in Chapter 11, Lymphatic Taping).

  If the injury is chronic, we may need to help stabilize the area or aid its movement. This is where taping combined with rehabilitation advice and exercises can really help, as the tape can help guide movements whilst the patient is strengthening and exercising the injured area. This can also help with neurological feedback and adaptive changes. Again, if the injury is chronic, commonly there are vascular changes in the area, therefore using tape to improve vascular dynamics can and will improve recovery.

1

- **Are you satisfied with the differential diagnosis?**
  Before you treat any area, be it with manual therapy, taping or any other modality, you must have an understanding of what the injury is. If you do not, you could either make the injury worse, or give the wrong support to the area. As we have already stressed, taping complements the skills you already have, and is not a treatment to be used on its own.

  In the case of taping someone before a sporting event or match, which you may not have examined or treated at this point, for safety and effectiveness you must examine and assess the patient before taping in order to ascertain how or what you want to achieve, and which tape is most appropriate for the task.

- **What was the injury onset?**
  Was it direct or indirect? Was it from trauma, repetitive strain, overuse or insidious factors? Each of these causes will affect how you manage the patient.

  Another consideration is your choice of tape colour, as this can have a psychological effect on the patient. For example, a brightly coloured k-tape could psychologically emphasize the injury more to the patient.

- **Are you familiar with the anatomy and function of the joint?**
  Knowledge of anatomy is key when using tape: you must have a good understanding of the structures under the skin to under-stand how taping can help. If you do not know the anatomy, how can you apply tape that is functionally going to change an area? Some people believe that knowing anatomy is all that's needed to begin taping an area. This is half true: yes knowing the anatomy and function of joints and action of muscles is important, but understanding the function, action and application of tapes is equally important. Relying solely on your knowledge of anatomy when taping can lead to further injury, hinder the healing process or produce no effect at all.

1

- **What do you want to achieve from taping?**
  There are two aspects to this question. First, is your goal to restrict movement or support a joint? Are you trying to help guide movement? Help in loading the joint or movement in the starting phase, or help decelerate or stabilize movement at the end phase? Help to improve fluid dynamics or even restrict them?
  Once you have ascertained what you want to achieve, the next question is which tape will help you achieve this? We hope to keep answering this throughout the book.

- **How much protection and support are required?**
  This is a little like the previous question regarding what you want to achieve, but there is a balance between protection and support, e.g., you can protect an area without giving restrictive support, and equally you can support movement or a ligament without necessarily giving it protection.

- **Do you have suitable materials?**
  Simply put, do you have the right tape for the right job, and do you have enough of it?

- **Will you further add to the injury if you tape at this stage?**
  This applies to both the acute and chronic phases. As discussed above, using a rigid or restrictive tape or technique during the acute inflammatory phase can compromise healing and recovery, and can be painful for the patient. You must also consider whether using tape to restrict or guide movements could cause further injury, either locally or indirectly to another part of the body (e.g., restricting movement in the ankle leading to issues with the knee). You may need to treat the injury first with manual therapy, exercise, or leave it alone and allow the area to rest and recover before using tape.

Important tips

- Never substitute treatment with taping: taping is a good addition to treatment but should never take the place of clinical assessment or therapy.
- Understanding the patient's job or sport helps you understand how to help and support movement, or in some circumstances restrict movement.
- Ensure the patient is aware of the restrictions or limitations of the taping, if there are any, before you tape or before they return to activity. Obviously when using rigid taping one of the objectives is to restrict movement, so clear communication is key.
- Never tape for no reason. As stated by Frett and Reilly (1994) unsuitable taping or taping for no reason could predispose an athlete to injury, or further aggravate an injury directly or indirectly elsewhere.

Contraindications and considerations for taping

Generally, taping is safe for everyone, from children to the elderly. Taping is not just for professional athletes, it can help anyone who needs it, but there are some conditions and situations where taping is not appropriate.

Allergic reactions to tapes in most circumstances will happen quickly, normally within 30 minutes after application. All the area that has been taped will be irritated, red, hot and itchy, and if left for long the skin will become raised. It's important to always inform the patient of this so they can identify the need to remove the tape if required. Therefore, as most treatment appointments last at least 30 minutes, if you or the patient are unsure if they will have a reaction to the tape, you can do a patch test by placing a small strip of tape on the patient at the beginning of the appointment.

1

Considerations
- allergies to tapes or plasters
- deep vein thrombosis (DVT) and phlebitis
- delicate skin, such as in the elderly
- skin has been shaved or waxed within the previous 24 hours.

Contraindications
- allergies to tapes or plasters
- skin conditions such as eczema, psoriasis and dermatitis
- cellulitis
- broken skin or wounds
- damaged skin, such as burns or sunburn
- infections
- compromised circulation and/or nerve supply, such as in diabetes and peripheral neuropathies
- lack of consent.

Pre-tape preparation

- The area to be taped should be clean and dry. When using tapes during sporting activities or events and the patient is already wet or sweaty, it is sometimes advisable to use a pre-tape spray to aid adhesion.
- Ideally the area should be hair free: ask patients to shave the area at least 24 hours before application, as this allows for the tape to adhere to the skin properly and reduces pain on removal (although with some rigid tape techniques you can use an under-wrap to aid removal, see Image 1.8).
- Do not use any lotions or oils to massage the area before taping as this will affect adhesion of the tape. Also ask the patient not to use lotions on the area themselves for the same reason.
- Always try to measure the area and assess how much tape you will need.

1

- For k-tape and biomechanical tape, the corners need to be rounded off (see Image 1.9) – this prevents the corners from snagging and helps the tape last longer (when you have a plaster on, it's the corners that get lifted and catch first).

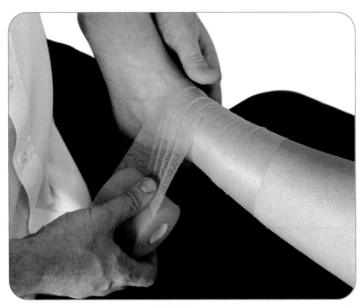

IMAGE 1.8

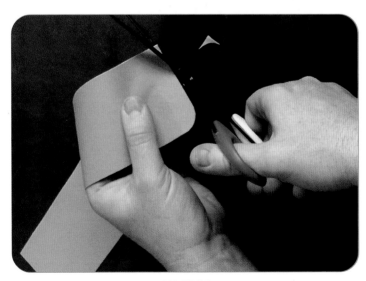

IMAGE 1.9

- It is also advisable that tapes do not get wet for at least an hour after application to help with adhesion. If the patient is intending on getting the tape wet sooner than this, it is advisable to use a pre-tape spray.

Overview of application

Traditional rigid tape methods use 'anchors' – strips of tape that are initially laid on the skin before beginning the main taping process (see Image 1.10).

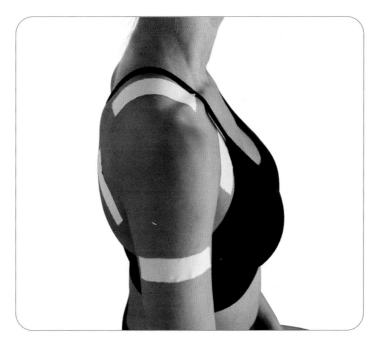

IMAGE 1.10

Anchors are used to avoid skin trauma: excessive pulling and loading on the skin leads to the skin breaking down, resulting in soreness, redness, splitting or blistering of the skin. Also, anchors give the tape that is subsequently applied an ideal area to adhere to, helping it last longer and giving better support.

Both k-tape and biomechanical tape do not require the use of anchors as they both 'self-anchor', i.e., when applying both these tapes, the end part does not have any stretch or traction placed on it. This prevents skin trauma as described above, and also helps with adhesion.

Complications from poor taping technique
Rigid tape

- Skin breakdown: Avoid excessive traction on the skin, commonly caused by unwinding and wrapping at the same time. This can also be caused by inadequate anchors.
- Skin blisters: Gaps and wrinkles may cause blisters, so care must be taken to avoid these. Wrinkles are commonly caused by using rigid tape that is too wide – 50 mm and occasionally 38 mm wide tapes (depending on the area) are difficult to use when negotiating angles or changes of direction around joints.
- Impairment of circulation: This can be the result of applying the tape too tightly, applying too many layers or not allowing a certain amount of give in the movement around the joint.

K-tape

- Skin blistering: This is the biggest issue resulting from poor technique with both k-tape and biomechanical tape. This can occur due to the anchors being either too short, or having tension applied to them during application. Anchors with k-tape should be approximately 5 cm, but in some circumstances in the book we will advise that long anchors should be used; in these cases the anchors should be approximately 8 cm or longer.

Biomechanical tape

- Skin blistering: Due to the stretch and recoil of biomechanical tape, poor technique commonly leads to traction blisters, which can be extreme. We generally advise that the self-anchors of biomechanical tape should be at least 6–8 cm in length, but in some areas we advise even longer, e.g., 10 cm plus.

Warning signs

It is extremely important to discuss these complications and reactions with your patient when taping, and to clearly communicate the signs and symptoms of circulation impairment:

- muscles that are sore, hurt more or are weak when using them
- pins and needles sensation
- cold fingers/toes
- increase in pain in the area
- numbness.

Skin blistering will feel sore and painful around the edges of the tape – patients will describe an uncomfortable pulling sensation on the skin and in some cases will show signs of skin blisters under the tape.

If a patient starts expressing any of the above, either take the tape off yourself if you are present or get the patient to take the tape off immediately.

Aftercare

Aftercare advice depends on what you are taping and the rationale behind it. However, the obvious applies every time:

- If you have a reaction to the tape – take it off.
- If the tape becomes painful or causes pain on movement – take it off.
- If it's uncomfortable – take it off.
- If you find it's restricting your circulation – take it off.
- If it's been on for longer than five days – take it off!

If you are using tape for an occasion such as a sporting event or match, you may just want to use the tape for a few hours before taking it off. On the other hand, you may wish the patient to leave the tape on for a few days, e.g., 2–4 days: if so, you will need to advise them regarding care of the tape. For example, if the tape becomes wet from bathing or swimming, they should pat the tape dry and not rub it with a towel, and **NEVER** use anything to heat dry the tape such as heat lamps or hair dryers. This can heat the glue in the tape, which can not only comprise the function of the glue but can heat it enough to burn the skin!

Tape removal

- Never leave tape on for longer than recommended: the maximum length of time is 4–5 days. I have heard stories of patients leaving tape on for weeks – resulting in the skin starting to grow into the tape! As you can imagine this can cause extreme complications when it comes to removing the tape.
- Never rip the tape off (although partners normally enjoy doing this!), as this can cause trauma and damage to the skin.
- When removing the tape, gently push the skin away from the tape rather than ripping the tape off, as this can damage the skin. In some circumstances no matter how you remove the tape it will be uncomfortable, but this is the least uncomfortable for the patient.
- You can also use tape remover spray which helps to disrupt the glue of the tape.
- Another tip is to suggest that your patient rubs either baby oil or massage oil into the tape 15–30 minutes before having a shower or bath as this helps denature the glue, and when washing to gently take the tape off.
- If you are going to use tape several times on a patient, we strongly advise that the skin has at least two days' rest between applications. Therefore, always remind your patient to remove the tape in adequate time to help the skin recover from the tape before applying again. The reason for this is that if you reapply tape over skin immediately after taking off, it is more prone to having a reaction to the tape either physiologically or mechanically.

References

Alahmari, K.A., Rengaramanujam, K., Reddy, R.S., Samuel, P.S., Tedla, J.S., Kakaraparthi, V.N. and Ahmad, I., 2020. The immediate and short-term effects of dynamic taping on pain, endurance, disability, mobility and kinesiophobia in individuals with chronic non-specific low back pain: a randomized controlled trial. *PLoS One, 15*(9), e0239505.

Artioli, D.P. and Bertolini, G.R.F., 2014. Kinesio taping: application and results on pain: systematic review. *Fisioterapia e Pesquisa,* 21, 94–99.

Bérdi, M., Köteles, F., Hevesi, K., Bárdos, G. and Szabo, A., 2015. Elite athletes' attitudes towards the use of placebo-induced performance enhancement in sports. *European Journal of Sport Science, 15*(4), 315–321

Chan, M.C.E., Wee, J.W.J. and Lim, M.H., 2017. Does kinesiology taping improve the early postoperative outcomes in anterior cruciate ligament reconstruction? A randomized controlled study. *Clinical Journal of Sport Medicine, 27*(3), 260–265.

Cimino, S.R., Beaudette, S.M. and Brown, S.H., 2018. Kinesio taping influences the mechanical behaviour of the skin of the low back: a possible pathway for functionally relevant effects. *Journal of Biomechanics, 67,* 150–156.

Clifford, A.M., Dillon, S., Hartigan, K., O'Leary, H. and Constantinou, M., 2020. The effects of McConnell patellofemoral joint and tibial internal rotation limitation taping techniques in people with patellofemoral pain syndrome. *Gait & Posture, 82,* 266–272.

Cochrane, M.E., Nkuna, F.S. and Dawood, M.A., 2023. The short-term effect of kinesio tape application on running speed, agility and plyometric performance in amateur soccer players. *South African Journal for Research in Sport, Physical Education & Recreation, 45*(1), 28–38.

Cook, J.L. and Purdam, CR., 2009. Is tendon pathology a continuum? A pathology model to explain the clinical presentation of load-induced tendinopathy. *British Journal of Sports Medicine, 43*(6), 409–416.

Cotterell, E. 1885. On some common injuries to limbs; Their treatment and after-treatment, including bone setting (so called). HK Lewis, London.

Csapo, R. and Alegre, L.M., 2015. Effects of Kinesio® taping on skeletal muscle strength: a meta-analysis of current evidence. *Journal of Science and Medicine in Sport, 18*(4), 450–456.

de Almeida Lins, C.A., Neto, F.L., de Amorim, A.B.C., de Brito Macedo, L. and Brasileiro, J.S., 2013. Kinesio Taping® does not alter neuromuscular performance of femoral quadriceps or lower limb function in healthy subjects: randomized, blind, controlled, clinical trial. *Manual Therapy, 18*(1), 41–45.

Frett, T.A. and Reilly, T.J., 1994. In: Mellion, M.B. (ed). *Sports Medicine Secrets.* Philadelphia: Hanley and Belfus; pp. 339–342.

Gatt, I.T., Allen, T. and Wheat, J., 2023. Effects of using rigid tape with bandaging techniques on wrist joint motion during boxing shots in elite male athletes. *Physical Therapy in Sport, 61,* 82–90.

Genc, A., Çelik, S.U., Genc, V., Öztuna, D. and Tur, B.S., 2019. The effects of cervical kinesiotaping on neck pain, range of motion, and disability in patients following thyroidectomy: a randomized, double-blind, sham-controlled clinical trial. *Turkish Journal of Medical Sciences, 49*(4), 1185–1191.

1

Gibney V. 1893. *The Modern Treatment of the Sprained Ankle.* The New York Polyclinic, pp. 3–6.

Hörmann, J., Vach, W., Jakob, M., Seghers, S. and Saxer, F., 2020. Kinesiotaping for postoperative oedema – what is the evidence? A systematic review. *BMC Sports Science, Medicine and Rehabilitation, 12*(1), 1–14.

Huang, T.Z. and Kim, S.Y., 2020. The effectiveness of upper limb offload dynamic taping technique on scapular muscles activation during elevation in healthy subjects. *Physical Therapy Korea, 27*(2), 93–101.

Kase, K., 1994. *Illustrated Kinesio-Taping,* 2nd edition. Tokyo, Japan: Ken'i-kai Information; pp. 6–9, 73.

Kase, K., 2003. *Clinical Therapeutic Applications of the Kinesio® Taping Method.* Albuquerque.

Kase, K. 2003. *Illustrated Kinesio Taping.* Tokyo, Japan: Ken'i-kai Information; pp. 6–12.

Kim, D.H. and Lee, Y., 2023. Effect of dynamic taping versus kinesiology taping on pain, foot function, balance, and foot pressure in 3 groups of plantar fasciitis patients: a randomized clinical study. *Medical Science Monitor, 29,* e941043–1.

Luo, W.H. and Li, Y., 2021. Current evidence does support the use of KT to treat chronic knee pain in short term: a systematic review and meta-analysis. *Pain Research and Management, 2021,* 5516389.

Maggi, L., Celletti, C., Mazzarini, M., Blow, D. and Camerota, F., 2022. Neuromuscular taping for chronic non-specific low back pain: a randomized single-blind controlled trial. *Aging Clinical and Experimental Research, 34*(5), 1171–1177.

McNeill, W. and Pedersen, C., 2016. Dynamic tape. Is it all about controlling load? *Journal of Bodywork and Movement Therapies, 20*(1), 179–188.

Mine, K., Nakayama, T., Milanese, S. and Grimmer, K., 2018. Effects of Kinesio tape on pain, muscle strength and functional performance: a systematic review of Japanese language literature. *Physical Therapy Reviews, 23*(2), pp.108–115.

Montalvo, A.M., Cara, E.L. and Myer, G.D., 2014. Effect of kinesiology taping on pain in individuals with musculoskeletal injuries: systematic review and meta-analysis. *The Physician and Sportsmedicine, 42*(2), 48–57.

Nichols, D.T., Robinson, T.L. and Oranchuk, D.J., 2019. Kinesiology taping of the ankle does not improve dynamic balance in NCAA athletes. *Athletic Training & Sports Health Care, 11*(1), 10–18.

Shah, M., Julu, P.O.O., Monro, J.A., Coutinho, J., Ijeh, C. and Puri, B.K., 2018. Neuromuscular taping reduces blood pressure in systemic arterial hypertension. *Medical Hypotheses, 116,* 30–32.

Shim, J.Y., Lee, H.R. and Lee, D.C., 2003. The use of elastic adhesive tape to promote lymphatic flow in the rabbit hind leg. *Yonsei Medical Journal, 44*(6), 1045–1052.

Singh, G., 2019. Athletic taping and its implications in sports. *International Journal on Integrated Education, 2*(4), 1–7.

Skirven T.M., Osterman A.L., Fedorczyk J.M. and Amadio, P.C., 2011. Elastic taping. In: *Rehabilitation of the Hand and Upper Extremity,* 6th edition. Elsevier, pp. 1529–1538.

Slomka, B., Rongies, W., Ruszczuk, P., Sierdzinski, J., Saganowska, D., Zdunski, S. and Worwag, M.E., 2018. Short-term effect of kinesiology taping on temperature distribution at the site of application. *Research in Sports Medicine, 26*(3), 365–380.

Song, J.Y., Park, S.H. and Lee, M.M., 2022. Comparison of the effects of dynamic taping and kinesio taping on endurance and fatigue of plantar flexor. *Journal of Korean Physical Therapy Science, 29*(1), 73–86.

Soslowsky, L.J., Thomopoulos, S., Esmail, A., Flanagan, C.L., Iannotti, J.P., Williamson, J.D. and Carpenter, J.E., 2002. Rotator cuff tendinosis in an animal model: role of extrinsic and overuse factors. *Annals of Biomedical Engineering, 30*, 1057–1063.

Tran, L., Makram, A.M., Makram, O.M., Elfaituri, M.K., Morsy, S., Ghozy, S., Zayan, A.H., Nam, N.H., Zaki, M.M.M., Allison, E.L. and Hieu, T.H., 2023. Efficacy of kinesio taping compared to other treatment modalities in musculoskeletal disorders: a systematic review and meta-analysis. *Research in Sports Medicine, 31*(4), 416–439.

Tu, S.J., Woledge, R.C. and Morrissey, D., 2016. Does 'Kinesio tape' alter thoracolumbar fascia movement during lumbar flexion? An observational laboratory study. *Journal of Bodywork and Movement Therapies, 20*(4), 898–905.

Upadhaya, S., Ram, C.S., Kumar, M. and Katiyar, N., (n.d.). Effect of kinesio taping and conventional physiotherapy on disability and pain in knee osteoarthritis. *Turkish Journal of Physiotherapy and Rehabilitation, 32*, 2.

Windisch, C., Brodt, S., Röhner, E. and Matziolis, G., 2017. Effects of Kinesio taping compared to arterio-venous Impulse System™ on limb swelling and skin temperature after total knee arthroplasty. *International Orthopaedics, 41*(2), 301–307. Erratum in: *International Orthopaedics*, 2017: *41*(4), 855.

Yam, M.L., Yang, Z., Zee, B.C.Y. and Chong, K.C., 2019. Effects of Kinesio tape on lower limb muscle strength, hop test, and vertical jump performances: a meta-analysis. *BMC Musculoskeletal Disorders, 20*, pp.1–12.

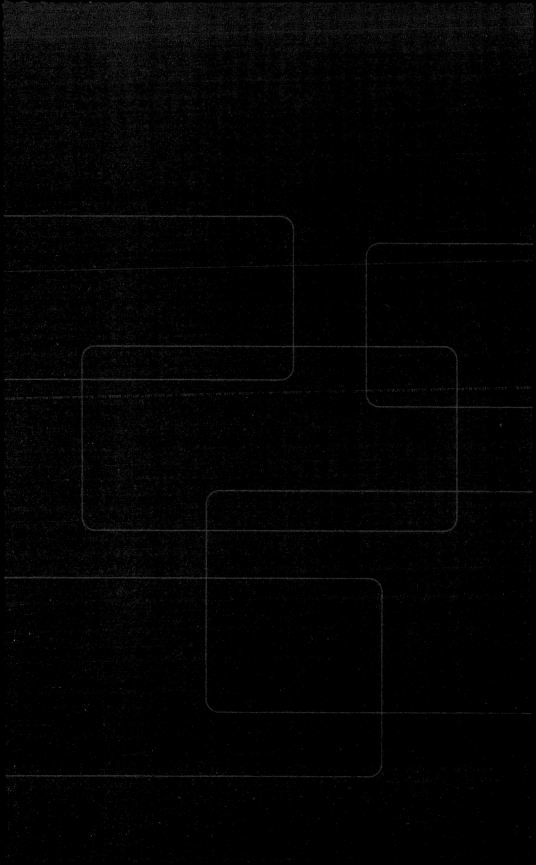

CHAPTER 2

Lumbar Spine

Research evidence

Research has shown that particularly in high-income countries, the incidence of acute low back pain is high, most often as a result of lifestyle factors that lead to obesity and decreased physical activity within the aging population. This incurs high costs worldwide due to the impact on quality of life and lost days due to inability to work (Oertel et al., 2024).

Patel and Shepherd (2024) discovered that between 2004 and 2019, there has been a steady increase in online health information-seeking behaviours for low back pain in the United Kingdom. This correlates to an increase in reported low back pain but also facilitates patients seeking early diagnosis and management advice.

Although more research needs to be done, the 4xT method shows promising signs of good outcomes and management of patients (Amstel et al., 2023; Van Amstel and Notan, 2023). The 4xT method consists of four components: Test (functional diagnostic test), Trigger (fascia tissue manipulations), Tape (elastic taping) and Train (exercise). This protocol is used in the management of low back pain and illustrates not only the benefit of having a clear protocol, but also how taping complements the treatment and rehabilitation of patients.

Grütters et al. (2023) suggest in their study that rigid taping may correct movement and improve performance during flexion-based tasks. In the same study they also suggested that t-tape may aid in improving proprioception and promote rehabilitation in the lumbar spine.

A systematic review by Nelson (2016) looked at the effects of k-tape on patients with chronic low back pain, and found that k-tape alone

2

was not a substitute for rehabilitation exercises, but the two combined produced favourable results. Aguilar-Ferrándiz et al. (2022) also found that the combination of rehabilitation exercises and k-taping showed improvements in pain, range of motion and a positive effect on mental health. Pakkir-Mohamed et al. (2023) concluded that physical therapy combined with the application of k-tape helped reduce pain and improve lumbar spine flexion, observed at two and six weeks post application. Sun and Lou (2021) also found that k-taping combined with rehabilitation exercises offered better therapeutic results with pain reduction and disability improvement compared with physical therapy alone in individuals with chronic low back pain.

K-taping can possibly influence postural control in participants with non-specific chronic low back pain according to research by Abbasi et al. in their study in 2018. They also found that k-tape decreased pain scores three days after application. Uzunkulaoğlu et al. (2018) found that k-tape produced statistically evident improvements in pain and range of movement short term, and improvements on range of movement long term. Wang et al. (2019) found with the aid of magnetic resonance elastography that k-taping had a positive effect on reducing stiffness in lumbar paraspinal muscles.

Pan et al. (2023) report that k-tape had an immediate and positive effect in reducing low back pain, but should not be used as a sole treatment modality for low back pain. This is also reflected in a study by Peñalver-Barrios et al. (2021), who observed short-term benefits in low back pain and also concluded that k-tape should only be used as a tool combined with rehabilitation and manual therapy.

Alahmari et al. (2020) found that biomechanical taping in chronic non-specific low back pain improved endurance in back extensors. They summarized that biomechanical tape helped control the process that led to back muscle fatigue and also helped aid movement through its range of motion. This is also reflected in a study by Jain et al., (2022) looking at the immediate effects of taping in sportspeople with non-specific low back pain. Penney (2019) also observed the off-loading effect of biomechanical taping in their study combining biomechanical taping and chiropractic manipulation for chronic mechanical low back pain.

Techniques

RIGID TAPING OF THE LUMBAR SPINE

▸ **Tape:** 38 mm rigid sports tape.

▸ **Position:** Patient seated in a semi-flexed position.

▸ **Actions:** To support the lumbar spine, and to reduce flexion in the lumbar spine.

▸ **Indications:** Acute low back pain; to limit flexion in the low back; disc herniation.

▸ **Instructions:** First, you will need to decide what levels you wish to restrict in the lower back and how much movement you wish to restrict. With an acute low back presentation, you should place the lower anchor over the sacrum at the level of S1. The upper anchor generally would be at the upper part of the lumbar spine at the level of L1 (Image 2.1).

As you place the anchors down, just lay them onto the skin, making sure you do not pull on the tape from one side to the other, as this can potentially cause skin blisters or an imbalance to your taping.

Now ask your patient to semi-bend forwards (this will depend on their mobility and also how much flexion you wish to restrict; the more flexed they are the less restrictive it is).

From the bottom anchor place a vertical strip of tape from the corner of the anchor directly superior to the upper anchor. Repeat this on the other side, thus taping a box to the patient's low back (Image 2.2).

To help reduce rotation and to support movement in the low back, lay two further strips superiorly from the corners of the lower anchors, but this time running diagonally to the opposite corners of the upper anchors (Image 2.3).

2

2

The vertical and diagonal strips can be repeated again with a 50% overlay. For more restriction into forward flexion, repeat with vertical strips over the first strip with an approximately 50% overlay. Repeat this on the other side. Keep repeating until you meet and overlay in the centre of the spine. If you require more restriction in rotation to one side, the taping can be repeated, but starting from the opposite corner of the lower anchor to the diagonally opposite corner. This would form an X on the vertical strips. This would restrict rotation to both sides and increase support to the lumbar spine. The application of tape can be increased until you are happy with the support given (Image 2.4).

Once finished, lay a second anchor strip over the original anchors securing the loose ends of the strips (Image 2.5).

As the patient straightens up, the slack in the tape will concertina with the skin. If your patient tries to go into lumbar flexion, the movement will be restricted (Image 2.6).

▸ **Tip:** With acute patients, rather than ask them to sit in a semi-flexed position, you can ask them to stand, bend forward and rest their hands on a table, work surface or treatment couch, thus supporting themselves more.

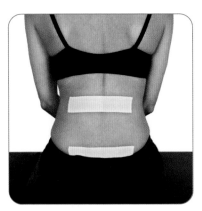

IMAGE 2.1

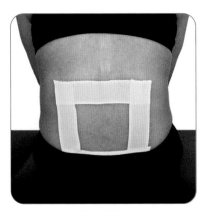

IMAGE 2.2

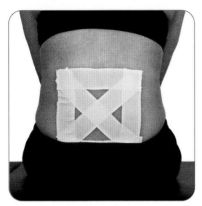

IMAGE 2.3

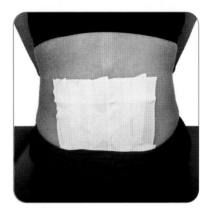

IMAGE 2.4

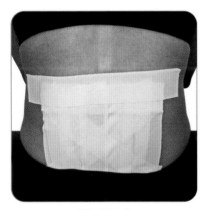

IMAGE 2.5

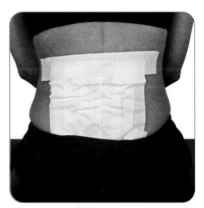

IMAGE 2.6

K-TAPING OF THE LUMBAR SPINE: STANDARD TECHNIQUE

▸ **Tape:** 50 mm k-tape.

▸ **Position:** Semi-flexed (slumped position).

▸ **Actions:** To provide increased circulation to the erector spinae and mild proprioceptive feedback.

▸ **Indications:** Returning to activity following spinal injury or inactivity.

▸ **Instructions:** This is possibly one of the most common k-tape techniques used for the lumbar spine. It provides minimal support but is primarily aimed at improving circulation to the erector spinae and surrounding tissues. It can also help to provide mild proprioceptive feedback.

First, cut two strips of identical length. With the first strip, place the anchor level with the base of the spine, over the bottom of the erector spinae. With a 50% stretch, lay the tape vertically along the erector spinae approximately 2–3 cm away from the midline. Lay the top anchor down onto the skin without any pre-stretch. The second strip is applied exactly the same way on the opposite side of the spine (Image 2.7).

A third horizontal strip can be placed on the area of spine that is painful or has suffered a past injury. This will provide mild proprioceptive feedback and support. Lay the centre length of the tape first, as this stops the tension on the tape pulling from one side to the other which could otherwise cause an imbalance in the pull of the tape from one side to the other (Image 2.8).

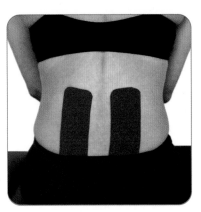

IMAGE 2.7

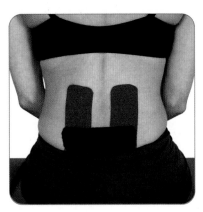

IMAGE 2.8

K-TAPING OF THE LUMBAR SPINE: PYRAMID TECHNIQUE

▸ **Tape:** 50 mm k-tape.

▸ **Position:** Semi-flexed (slumped position).

▸ **Actions:** To lift the tissues of the lower lumbar spine and provide support.

▸ **Indications:** Acute lower back pain.

▸ **Instructions:** With this technique we are using the rigid resistance of the k-tape as it does not stretch across the width of the tape. Cut three strips of k-tape at equal lengths and three strips of different lengths (approximately 10 cm, 13 cm and 15 cm long, depending on the size of the patient).

First, we are going to use the three different length strips. Lay the shortest strip below the segment you wish to support (e.g., if supporting L5/S1, place the short strip over the level of S1). Instead of placing the anchors first, we need to apply the centre piece of the tape first. Break off and remove the centre of the backing tape, apply a 50% stretch onto the tape and place directly onto the skin (Image 2.9). Placing the centre length of the tape first can help prevent pulling from one side to the other. Once the centre piece of the tape is applied, remove the backing paper from the anchors and lay them down with no stretch (Image 2.10).

This process is repeated with the middle strip with a 50% overlay superiorly to the first tape (Image 2.11). The middle tape should be over the level of the lumbar spine that requires the most support. The process is repeated again with the third longer strip, using a 50% overlay on the middle strip (Image 2.12). You should now have what resembles an upside-down pyramid on the lower back. Due to the lack of stretch along its width, the k-tape will produce some restriction of movement and support.

Now with the three identical length strips, take one strip and remove the backing off one end for your anchor, and place the anchor vertically and centrally over the base of your pyramid. With a 50% stretch, place the middle of the tape vertically over the spine and the end anchor with no stretch (Image 2.13).

Place the anchor of the second strip centrally over the first anchor, but at a 45-degree angle. With a 50% stretch, place the middle of the tape continuing at the 45-degree angle, and then lay the end anchor down with no stretch (Image 2.14). Repeat this process again for the third strip, with the bottom anchor centrally but at a 45-degree angle to the opposite side of the second tape. Repeat with a 50% stretch for the middle and place the top anchor with no stretch (Image 2.15).

Note: This technique uses multiple layers centrally over the same area giving focussed support to the area.

▸ **Tip:** If it's too uncomfortable for the patient to sit in a slumped position, ask your patient to stand and bend forwards, supporting themselves on a table or treatment couch. If your couch is adjustable in height, you can raise it or lower it to the desired height and control the amount of standing flexion in your patient's spine.

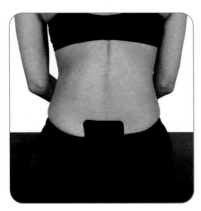

IMAGE 2.9

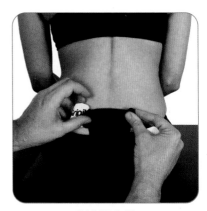

IMAGE 2.10

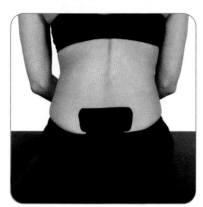

IMAGE 2.11

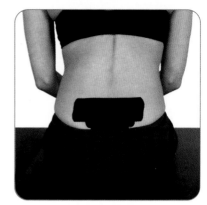

IMAGE 2.12

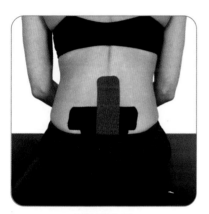

IMAGE 2.13

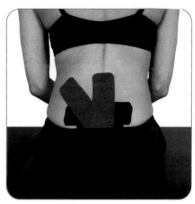

IMAGE 2.14

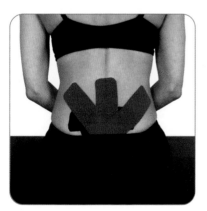

IMAGE 2.15

BIOMECHANICAL TAPING OF THE LUMBAR SPINE: ARROW TECHNIQUE

2

▶ **Tape:** 75 mm biomechanical tape.

▶ **Position:** Prone.

▶ **Actions:** To support the lower back into flexion and rotation.

▶ **Indications:** Recovering low back pain injury.

▶ **Instructions:** For this technique you will need four lengths of 75 mm biomechanical tape. With the first strip, place the inferior anchor over the lower portion of the erector spinae at the level of S1. Placing a small amount of tension on the tape, lay the middle of the tape directly vertical to the anchor over the erector spinae. With no tension, apply the superior anchor down and smooth the tape over. Repeat this action on the opposite side of the spine (Image 2.16).

Once you have completed both vertical strips, take one of the extra strips and place the lower anchor over the inferior anchor of the first. Lay the next strip at a 45-degree angle to the vertical strip going laterally. Place the anchor with no tension, then with a small amount of tension on the tape, place diagonally at 45 degrees to the vertical at the middle portion of the tape. Apply the upper anchor with no pre-stretch.

Repeat this on the opposite side, but as a mirrored reflection to the previous strip, running 45 degrees laterally. When this is completed, together the tapes should look like an arrow pointing down (Image 2.17).

▶ **Tip:** Do not go too central and place the vertical strips over the middle of the spine. You can just use the two vertical strips without the diagonal strips if you wish. You can also laminate the strips for extra tension and support.

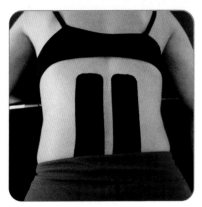
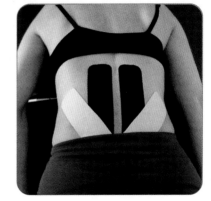

IMAGE 2.16   IMAGE 2.17

BIOMECHANICAL TAPING OF THE LUMBAR SPINE: CROSS TAPING TECHNIQUE

▸ **Tape:** 50 mm or 75 mm Active Tape.

▸ **Position:** Prone.

▸ **Actions:** To give support to the lower back, especially with flexion and rotation.

▸ **Indications:** Segmental lumbar support; disc herniation.

▸ **Instructions:** Cut four strips of biomechanical tape. Using the first strip, place the anchor at approximately 45 degrees to the vertical over the mid-lateral area of the upper buttock. Place one hand over the anchor slightly and push away at the same time. With a small amount of tension placed on the middle portion of the tape, cross over the spine superiorly in a diagonal direction. Apply and smooth the upper anchor onto the skin with no pre-stretch. Smooth the tape over, making sure of good adherence over the centre of the spine (Image 2.18).

Take the second strip of tape and place the lower anchor on the opposite mid-lateral buttock. Repeat the same process as the first strip with a small amount of pre-stretch on the middle section of the tape. The second strip will cross over the first forming an X on the lower back. The two tapes should cross at the level of the spine you wish to support the most (Image 2.19).

Repeat the same process as above with the third and fourth strips, but with a 50% overlay of the tapes (Image 2.20). This will provide maximum support at the level of the cross (Image 2.21).

▸ **Tip:** To get an idea of where you want to attach the tape, lay the tape over the area without taking the backing off, this way you can place and adjust to get the best idea of level and angle of the tape. The level where the tapes cross over can be brought higher or lower depending on the level needed for maximum support.

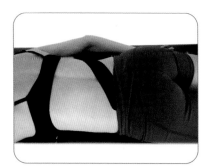

IMAGE 2.18

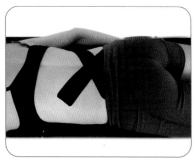

IMAGE 2.19

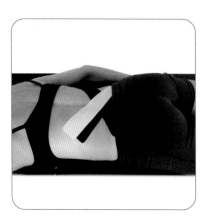

IMAGE 2.20

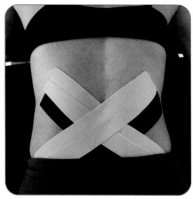

IMAGE 2.21

References

Abbasi, S., Rojhani-Shirazi, Z., Shokri, E. and San José, F.G.M., 2018. The effect of Kinesio Taping on postural control in subjects with non-specific chronic low back pain. *Journal of Bodywork and Movement Therapies, 22*(2), 487–492.

Aguilar-Ferrándiz, M.E., Matarán-Peñarrocha, G.A., Tapia-Haro, R.M., Castellote-Caballero, Y., Martí-García, C. and Castro-Sánchez, A.M. (2022). Effects of a supervised exercise program in addition to electrical stimulation or kinesio taping in low back pain: a randomized controlled trial. *Scientific Reports, 12*(1), 11430.

Alahmari, K.A., Rengaramanujam, K., Reddy, R.S., Samuel, P.S., Tedla, J.S., Kakaraparthi, V.N. and Ahmad, I., 2020. The immediate and short-term effects of dynamic taping on pain, endurance, disability, mobility and kinesiophobia in individuals with chronic non-specific low back pain: a randomized controlled trial. *PLoS One, 15*(9), e0239505.

Amstel, R.V., Noten, K., Malone, S. and Vaes, P., 2023. Fascia tissue manipulations in chronic low back pain: a pragmatic comparative randomized clinical trial of the 4xT Method® and exercise therapy. *Life, 14*(1), 7.

Grütters, K., Narciss, S., Beaudette, S.M. and Oppici, L., 2023. Reducing lumbar flexion in a repetitive lifting task: comparison of leukotape and kinesio tape and their effect on lumbar proprioception. *Applied Sciences, 13*(10), 5908.

Jain, P., Misra, A. and Pal, A., 2022. The immediate effects of dynamic taping on endurance, pain, disability and mobility in sports person with non-specific low back pain. *Indian Journal of Applied Research, 12*(4), 77–79.

Nelson, N.L., 2016. Kinesio taping for chronic low back pain: a systematic review. *Journal of Bodywork and Movement Therapies, 20*(3), 672–681.

Oertel, J., Sharif, S., Zygourakis, C. and Sippl, C., 2024. Acute low back pain: epidemiology, etiology, and prevention: WFNS Spine Committee recommendations. *World Neurosurgery, X*, 100313.

Pakkir Mohamed, S.H., Al Amer, H.S. and Nambi, G., 2023. The effectiveness of kinesio taping and conventional physical therapy in the management of chronic low back pain: a randomized clinical trial. *Clinical Rheumatology, 42*(1), 233–244.

Pan, L., Li, Y., Gao, L., Sun, Y., Li, M., Zhang, X., Wang, Y. and Shi, B., 2023. Effects of kinesio taping for chronic nonspecific low back pain: a systematic review and meta-analysis. *Alternative Therapies in Health and Medicine, 29*(6), 68–76.

Patel, H. and Shepherd, T.A., 2024. Online health information-seeking behaviours for low back pain in the United Kingdom: analysis of data from Google trends and the Global Burden of Disease Study, 2004–2019. *International Health*, ihae020. doi:10.1093/inthealth/ihae020.

Peñalver-Barrios, M.L., Lisón, J.F., Ballester-Salvador, J., Schmitt, J., Ezzedinne-Angulo, A., Arguisuelas, M.D. and Doménech, J., 2021. A novel (targeted) kinesio taping application on chronic low back pain: randomized clinical trial. *PLoS One, 16*(5), e0250686.

Penney, M., 2019. The efficacy of chiropractic manipulation and dynamic taping of the lumbar spine in isolation and then as a combined therapy in the treatment of chronic mechanical lower back pain (Doctoral dissertation, University of Johannesburg (South Africa)).

Sun, G. and Lou, Q., 2021. The efficacy of kinesio taping as an adjunct to physical therapy for chronic low back pain for at least two weeks: a systematic review and meta-analysis of randomized controlled trials. *Medicine, 100*(49), e28170.

Uzunkulaoğlu, A., Aytekin, M.G., Ay, S. and Ergin, S., 2018. The effectiveness of kinesio taping on pain and clinical features in chronic non-specific low back pain: a randomized controlled clinical trial. *Turkish Journal of Physical Medicine and Rehabilitation, 64*(2), 126.

van Amstel, R.N. and Noten, K., 2023. Unlocking pain relief for chronic low back pain: the potential of the 4xT Method®: a dual case study analysis. *The American Journal of Case Reports, 24*, e939284–1.

Wang, C.K., Fang, Y.H.D., Lin, L.C., Lin, C.F., Kuo, L.C., Chiu, F.M. and Chen, C.H., 2019. Magnetic resonance elastography in the assessment of acute effects of kinesio taping on lumbar paraspinal muscles. *Journal of Magnetic Resonance Imaging, 49*(4), 1039–1045.

CHAPTER 3

Thoracic Spine and Ribs

Research evidence

In old martial arts movies, you would often see the hero getting injured and having their ribs heavily strapped with rigid tape to protect them. Unfortunately, this has been generally found to be not recommended as a treatment approach nowadays. The reason being that rigid taping of the chest and over the ribs can restrict breathing and compromise rib function, potentially leading to complications such as pneumonia or reduced lung function. However, there is no such evidence of harmful consequences from biomechanical taping of the ribs, and the use of k-tape has been found to be beneficial following rib trauma and fracture.

K-tape is very effective in the recovery and treatment of MMA fighters, boxers and athletes who particate in throwing sports and who get side strains and intercostal strains. This is supported by studies such as that by Abd Al Raheem et al. (2022) that showed the importance of the concurrent application of k-tape with inspiratory muscle training in athletes in improving muscle pressure. Bakker et al. (2022) found that uncomplicated traumatic shoulder and chest wall injuries responded better with the use of k-tape combined with standard care including analgesic care and slings, than standard care alone. Ökmen et al. (2019) observed that patients with stable chronic obstructive pulmonary disease (COPD) showed better improvement in respiratory function when routine medical treatment was combined with k-tape than treatment alone. The use of k-tape over a six-week period can also benefit chest expansion and strength (Thongchote et al., 2023).

There is also good evidence supporting the use of k-tape following rib fractures. Sareen et al. (2015) discovered a significant decrease in pain while deep breathing and coughing, when comparing the use of kinesiology taping before and after application for treating undisplaced rib fracture pain. Akça et al. (2020) and Cakmak et al. (2021) also observed that combined k-tape and NSAID therapy in the treatment of uncomplicated rib fractures was more effective in reducing pain compared to NSAIDs alone. Imperatori et al. (2016) also reported that k-tape was a safe and effective auxiliary technique for chest pain with patients following a lung lobectomy.

In regards biomechanical taping to ribs there is no evidence to date but considering the elastic support and restriction of biomechanical taping, k-tape is the best option in regards treating rib injuries.

In the treatment of posture, Rayjade et al. (2020) found that k-taping was effective in reducing pain and improving posture in patients with upper cross syndrome, with Chaudhuri et al. (2023) also reporting that exercise combined with the use of k-tape was beneficial in the same setting. Vinken and Heinen (2015) also state that k-tape is effective in immediate and mid-term posture control. The important finding of these and other studies regarding postural support and k-tape, is that k-tape is not an effective stand-alone treatment, but when combined with exercises, produces more effective results than exercise alone.

Similar results have been reported with biomechanical taping, including improvement of shoulder range of movement and upper body posture following acromioplasty and rotator cuff repair surgery (Park and Kim, 2018), improvement in back muscle endurance and postural support (Alahmari et al., 2020), and deloading of trapezius, pain reduction and improvement in posture (Yoon and Kim, 2022).

Techniques

K-TAPING FOR THE THORACIC SPINE: RIB PAIN

▶ **Tape:** 50 mm k-tape.

▸ **Position:** Side-lying with the shoulder abducted, or sitting and leaning to the side with the shoulder abducted.

▸ **Actions:** To reduce pain over the intercostal muscles and improve chest expansion.

▸ **Indications:** Intercostal pain/side strain.

▸ **Instructions:** Cut two strips of tape the same length. With your patient stretching the side affected, palpate for the angle of the ribs (Image 3.1). The area that you are taping is over the intercostal space *between* the ribs and not over the ribs.

    Starting from the outer edge of the erector spinae, place the anchor of the tape with a 50–75% stretch to the middle section of the tape. Smooth the tape along the angle of the ribs over the intercostal space. Continue until you reach the midline of the rib and apply the anchor (Image 3.2). Repeat the procedure and apply to the next intercostal space (Image 3.3).

    Apply a third piece of k-tape and stretch (50–75%) vertically along the midline of the intercostal tapes (Image 3.4).

▸ **Tip:** As you are positioning the tape, place a finger in the intercostal space for a visual reference.

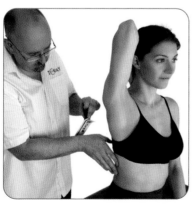 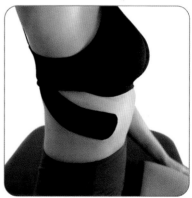

IMAGE 3.1   IMAGE 3.2

3

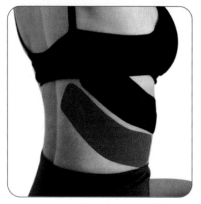

IMAGE 3.3

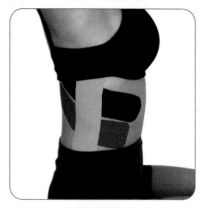

IMAGE 3.4

K-TAPING FOR THE THORACIC SPINE:
TRAPEZIUS AND RHOMBOID PAIN

▸ **Tape:** 50 mm k-tape.

▸ **Position:** Patient in a neutral position.

▸ **Actions:** To lift the skin over the trapezius and rhomboids.

▸ **Indications:** Localized muscle tension.

▸ **Instructions:** Cut two strips of tape the same length. Cut both down the middle, creating Y-strips, leaving approximately 8–9 cm at the end for the anchor. Apply the anchor over the medial periscapular area. Starting with the section of tape closest to the spine, stretch the tape 50–75% and apply over the skin towards the neck. Place your anchor on the base of the neck over the trapezius. With the second section of tape, repeat the same process but aim towards the middle of the trapezius (Image 3.5).

    Using the second strip, place the anchor over the upper portion of the deltoid. Stretch (50–75%) one section over the top of the shoulder and trapezius (if cut a little long, go over the base of the neck towards the opposite shoulder). With the second section of the tape stretched 50–75%, apply 1–2 cm below the first strip in the same direction (Image 3.6).

▸ **Tip:** This taping can be applied to both sides of the body.

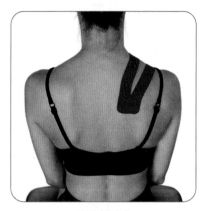
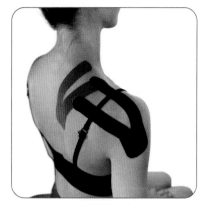

IMAGE 3.5   IMAGE 3.6

K-TAPING FOR THE THORACIC SPINE: MID THORACIC PAIN

▸ **Tape:** 50 mm k-tape.

▸ **Position:** Patient in a neutral position.

▸ **Actions:** To improve fluid dynamics to the periscapular muscles.

▸ **Indications:** Mid thoracic pain.

▸ **Instructions:** Cut a long strip of k-tape and cut down the centre of the tape leaving a broad anchor at the base. With the first section of tape, with an approximately 50–75% stretch to the middle of the tape, lay the tape over the thoracic erector spinae and up and over the midline of the upper trapezius. With no stretch, smooth the end anchor down to the skin. Repeat the same process with the second section on the opposite side (Image 3.7).

A vertical strip of tape can be placed horizontally to help keep the scapula retracted. To do this, find the middle of a strip of tape and break the backing, take the middle of the tape and place without stretch of the spine. Ask your patient to retract their shoulders and with a 50% stretch, apply the tape horizontally to the scapula. Repeat this on the other side. This can be done with either k-tape or biomechanical tape (some people may find using biomechanical tape provides better support). The vertical strip is placed in the same way as shown in Image 3.11.

▶ **Tip:** Starting from the middle and stretching the horizontal strip to either side prevents excessive pull to one side or the other. Also, the anchors of the horizontal strip must stick over the edge of the scapula to be effective.

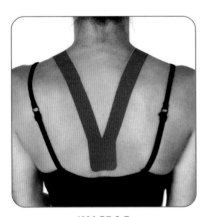

IMAGE 3.7

BIOMECHANICAL TAPING FOR THE THORACIC SPINE: POSTURAL SUPPORT

▸ **Tape:** 50 mm biomechanical tape.

▸ **Position:** Patient in a neutral position.

▸ **Actions:** To support posture.

▸ **Indications:** Protracted shoulders and poor posture.

▸ **Instructions:** Cut two pieces of tape the same length. With a long anchor, apply the tape over the patient's chest, angling towards the tip of the shoulder. Ask your patient to retract their shoulders. Smooth the tape over the angle of the shoulder (Image 3.8). With your patient keeping their shoulders retracted, take the slack out of the tape and smooth the tape down running diagonally down over the scapula and across the spine. Repeat the same process on the opposite side (Images 3.9 and 3.10).

Using a 100 mm strip of biomechanical tape, find the middle of a strip of tape and break the backing, take the middle of the tape and apply it without stretch of the spine. Ask your patient to retract their shoulders and lay the tape horizontally to the scapula. Repeat this on the other side (Image 3.11).

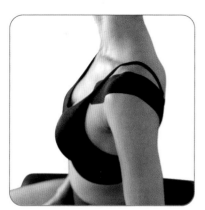

IMAGE 3.8

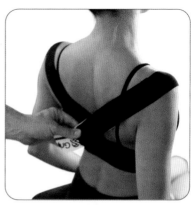

IMAGE 3.9

3

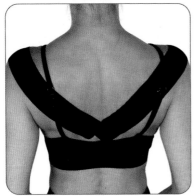

IMAGE 3.10

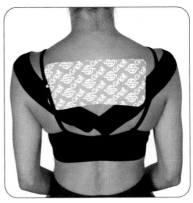

IMAGE 3.11

▸ **Tips:** Make sure you use long anchors over the chest to prevent skin blisters on sensitive chest skin.

Starting from the middle and stretching the horizontal strip to either side prevents excessive pull to one side or the other. Also, the anchors of the horizontal strip must stick over the edge of the scapula to be effective.

When negotiating around bras and clothing, keep the backing paper on the tape and take off a small part at a time, allowing you to tuck the tape under clothing without getting the tape stuck together.

References

Abd Al Raheem, A.A., El Nahas, N.G. and Ibrahim, E.M., 2022. Concurrent effect of inspiratory muscles training and kinesio taping on inspiratory muscles pressure in athletes. *International Journal of Thin Films Science and Technology, 11* (S1), 23–27.

Akça, A.H., Şaşmaz, M.İ. and Kaplan, Ş., 2020. Kinesiotaping for isolated rib fractures in the emergency department. *The American Journal of Emergency Medicine, 38*(3), 638–640.

Alahmari, K.A., Rengaramanujam, K., Reddy, R.S., Samuel, P.S., Tedla, J.S., Kakaraparthi, V.N. and Ahmad, I., 2020. The immediate and short-term effects of dynamic taping on pain, endurance, disability, mobility and kinesiophobia in individuals with chronic non-specific low back pain: a randomized controlled trial. *PLoS One, 15*(9), e0239505.

Bakker, M.E., Bon, V.J., Huybrechts, B.P., Scott, S., Zwartsenburg, M.M. and Goslings, J.C., 2022. Kinesiotaping in the emergency department: the effect of kinesiotaping on acute pain due to uncomplicated traumatic injury of the shoulder or chest wall. A pilot study. *The American Journal of Emergency Medicine*, *58*, 197–202.

Cakmak, M., Aydin, S. and Balci, A.E., 2021. The comparison of analgesics and kinesiological taping in rib fractures. *Indian Journal of Surgery*, *83*(S1), 190–194.

Chaudhuri, S., Chawla, J.K. and Phadke, V., 2023. Physiotherapeutic interventions for upper cross syndrome: a systematic review and meta-analysis. *Cureus*, *15*(9).

Imperatori, A., Grande, A., Castiglioni, M., Gasperini, L., Faini, A., Spampatti, S., Nardecchia, E., Terzaghi, L., Dominioni, L. and Rotolo, N., 2016. Chest pain control with kinesiology taping after lobectomy for lung cancer: initial results of a randomized placebo-controlled study. *Interactive Cardiovascular and Thoracic Surgery*, *23*(2), 223–230.

Ökmen, B.M., Dikiş, Ö.Ş., Ökmen, K., Altan, L. and Yildiz, T., 2019. Investigation of the effect of kinesiotaping on the respiratory function and depression in male patients with chronic obstructive pulmonary disease: a prospective, randomized, controlled, and single-blind study. *The Aging Male*, *23*(5), 648–654.

Park, S.J. and Kim, S.Y., 2018. The effect of scapular dynamic taping on pain, disability, upper body posture and range of motion in the postoperative shoulder. *Korean Society of Physical Medicine*, *13*(4), 149–162.

Rayjade, A., Yadav, T., Chintamani, R. and Joshi, N., 2020. Comparative effectiveness of kinesio taping and IFT in upper cross syndrome: a randomized clinical trial. *Indian Journal of Forensic Medicine & Toxicology*, *14*(3), 127–132.

Sareen, A., Jain, P. and Pagare, V., 2015. Immediate effect of kinesiology taping in treating undisplaced rib fracture pain. *Journal of Musculoskeletal Research*, *18*(02), 1550010.

Thongchote, K., Sangchuchuenjit, C., Vichaichotikul, W., Choosaranon, N., Kulsiri, N., Lopansri, P., Jaysrichai, T. and Lapmanee, S., 2023. The functional correction of forward shoulder posture with kinesiotape improves chest mobility and inspiratory muscle strength: a randomized controlled trial. *Annals of Applied Sport Science*, *11*(2), 0–0.

Vinken, P.M. and Heinen, T., 2015. Immediate and mid-term effects of elastic taping on gymnast's postural control performance during a handstand. *Baltic Journal of Health and Physical Activity*, *7*(4), 7.

Yoon, S.W. and Kim, S.Y., 2022. Effects of upper trapezius inhibition dynamic taping on pain, function, range of motion, psychosocial status, and posture of the neck in patients with chronic neck pain. *Physical Therapy Korea*, *29*(1), 1–10.

CHAPTER 4

Shoulder

Research evidence

Shoulder injuries are extremely common in sports, especially in over-use sports such as volleyball, basketball, baseball and handball (Kraan et al., 2019), and in impact sports such as rugby (Partner et al., 2022), American football (Anderson et al., 2021) and Australian rules football (Schwab, 2020). Hodgetts et al. (2021) found that the prevalence of shoulder pain generally increases in physically active occupations after the age of 50, especially when compared to sedentary occupations. Management and return to work and play can be complicated, as patients will either return back to the same work or sport that caused the issues in the first place (Cools et al., 2021). Therefore, our management strategy is not only how to treat and manage the symptoms, but also how to best prepare the patient to return to activity. Giving patients the right rehabilitation tools is key, and supporting and protecting the joint with the appropriate taping or strapping is also essential (Olsen and Gregory, 2023).

In their 2012 study, McConnell et al. reported that rigid sports taping increased the protection of shoulder injuries in athletes, and also improved scapular muscle control. Dewir et al. (2023) found rigid taping effective in improving functional disability and pain in subacromial impingement syndrome. Ozer et al. (2018) looked at the effects of rigid and k-taping on shoulder and scapular regional pain in overhead athletes, and found that both helped improve scapular dyskinesis. A further systematic review by Turgut et al. (2023) also found that taping combined with rehabilitation was effective in the treatment of shoulder injuries in overhead athletes.

In a study examining pain and disability, exercise combined with k-taping showed significant improvement when compared with exercise alone (Ghozy et al., 2020). In their study of the effects of k-taping on adhesive capsulitis, Thalagala and Sankalpani (2023) found that taping alone was not statistically effective, but produced better results when combined with treatment and rehabilitation compared with treatment alone. Saracoglu et al. (2018) also found that k-tape was an effective add-on to treatments such as rehabilitation, electrotherapy and manual therapy. Studies by Letafatkar et al. (2021) and Kim et al. (2022) found that adding k-tape to rehabilitation improved clinical outcomes in patients with shoulder impingement syndrome and shoulder pain in tennis players, respectively. Snodgrass et al. (2018) state that rehabilitation should be introduced immediately after tape has been applied to derive maximum benefit.

Yang et al. (2018) studied the effect of k-taping on hemiplegic shoulder pain and found improvements in pain and muscle activity immediately, and again at four weeks. These findings are reflected in studies by Deng (2021), Tan (2022) and Wang (2022). Tudini et al. (2023) reported that k-tape offered improvements in pain and function in patients with hypermobile Ehlers-Danlos syndrome and shoulder pain.

A 2023 study by Huang et al. found that biomechanical tape reduced direction-specific shoulder fatigue in amateur baseball players. Park and Kim (2018) studied the effect of biomechanical taping in patients who had undergone acromioplasty and rotator cuff repair surgery, and found that biomechanical taping was effective in improving shoulder disability and range of movement. Further studies have confirmed the effectiveness of biomechanical taping for improved shoulder proprioception (Park et al., 2020) and in facilitating rehabilitation exercises by improving range of movement and pain in patients with subacromial impingement syndrome (Göktaş et al., 2022).

Techniques

RIGID TAPING OF THE SHOULDER: SHOULDER SUPPORT

▸ **Tape:** 38 mm/50 mm rigid sports tape.

▸ **Position:** Shoulder in an abducted position with the hand on the hip.

▸ **Actions:** To stabilize the acromioclavicular and glenohumeral joint; limit end range of movement; particularly useful with sports that take impact through the shoulder, e.g., rugby, American football, martial arts and other high-impact sports.

▸ **Indications:** Instability of acromioclavicular and glenohumeral joint; early-stage dislocation of the glenohumeral joint.

▸ **Instructions:** Apply four anchors: 1. mid trapezius, 2. deltoid tuberosity, 3. lower angle of scapula (at a slight angle), 4. mid chest level (at slight angle). Each anchor should be between 10 and 15 cm, depending on size of patient (Images 4.1 and 4.2).

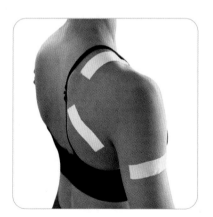

IMAGE 4.1

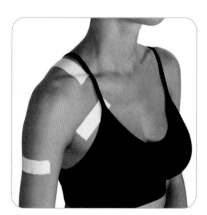

IMAGE 4.2

Without any pull through the tape, apply tape from the corner of the trapezius down to the corner of the anchor below on the same side. Repeat this on the opposite corner, thus forming a box shape (Image 4.3).

Then apply tape from one corner of the anchor on the trapezius down to the opposite corner of the anchor over the deltoid tuberosity. This is then repeated from the other corner of the anchor over the trapezius to the opposite corner of the lower anchor (Image 4.4). These can be repeated several times with a 25–50% overlay on the previous strip until the anchors are covered (Image 4.5).

If you want to add extra protection to the upper shoulder and acromioclavicular joint, padding can be applied over the acromioclavicular joint (not shown) and the previous step is repeated to give the shoulder the maximum support and protection.

This process is repeated with the chest and scapula anchors going from opposite corners initially twice and then applying strips with 25–50% overlay going straight over from anchor to anchor (Images 4.6 and 4.7). Be careful not to pull the tape over the trapezius and then go from anchor to anchor, as this will compress and apply pressure down on the shoulder and be uncomfortable.

To finish, reapply the tape over the original anchors (Image 4.8), or for maximum adhesion, wrap completely around the arm with the final anchor and also completely around the torso.

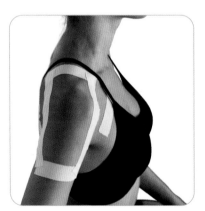

IMAGE 4.3

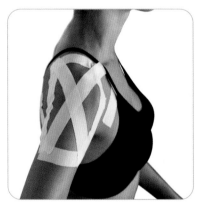

IMAGE 4.4

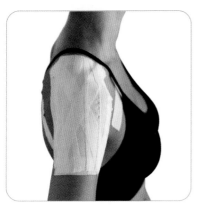

IMAGE 4.5

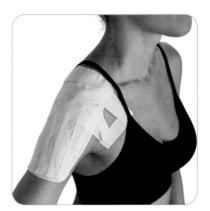

IMAGE 4.6

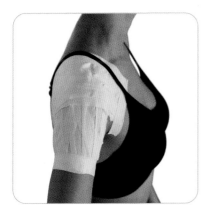

IMAGE 4.7

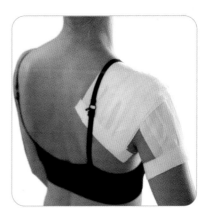

IMAGE 4.8

K-TAPING OF THE SHOULDER: ROTATOR CUFF

▸ **Tape:** 50 mm k-tape.

▸ **Position:** Upper extremity should be initially resting to the side of the body.

▸ **Actions:** To aid proprioception of the shoulder; give gentle support for the glenohumeral and acromioclavicular joint; improve fluid dynamics of the deltoid muscle.

▸ **Indications:** To aid fluid mechanics following injury or impact to shoulder; may help with supraspinatus, infraspinatus and biceps brachii tendinopathy.

▸ **Instructions:** Cut down the centre of a piece of tape leaving 8–9 cm at the end for the anchor. Apply the anchor with no stretch over the deltoid tuberosity, or slightly below. Before applying the anterior strip, ask your patient to externally rotate their shoulder. With a 50% stretch on the tape, apply along the anterior border of the middle head of the deltoid, running up and over the shoulder; once this has been done, smooth down the anchor (Image 4.9). The tape application is repeated for the posterior border of the middle head of the deltoid (Image 4.10).

This can be repeated for the anterior and posterior borders of the anterior and posterior heads of the deltoid for maximum effect (Image 4.11).

This can be done in any order. If desired, focus on an individual part of the deltoid.

A horizontal strip is then applied just above the deltoid tuberosity with a 50% stretch, placing the anterior anchor onto the chest and the posterior anchor onto the scapula (Image 4.12). This will give a compressive support to the shoulder, thus giving some support to the glenohumeral joint.

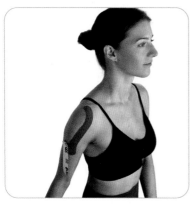

IMAGE 4.9

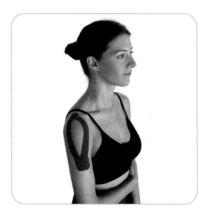

IMAGE 4.10

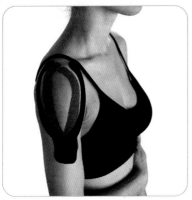

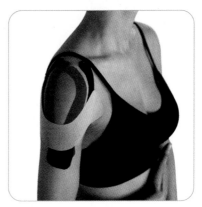

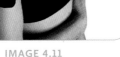

IMAGE 4.11   IMAGE 4.12

4

K-TAPING OF THE SHOULDER:
ACROMIOCLAVICULAR JOINT

▶ **Tape:** 50 mm k-tape.

▶ **Position:** Arm and shoulder in a neutral position.

▶ **Actions:** To help support the acromioclavicular joint.

▶ **Indications:** Acromioclavicular joint sprain.

▶ **Instructions:** Cut three short pieces of k-tape of the same length. Apply the first strip directly over the joint line of the acromioclavicular joint, with an approximately 75% stretch to the middle portion (Image 4.13). The next two strips are laid at 45 degrees each way to the first, creating a star pattern over the acromioclavicular joint, with 75% stretch to the middle portions (Images 4.14 and 4.15).

▶ **Tip:** Palpate for the joint line before taping as the acromioclavicular joint is a very variable joint. This technique can also be used with biomechanical tape to give a more supportive effect to the area.

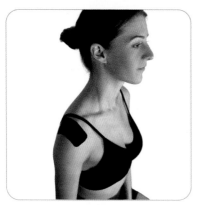

IMAGE 4.13

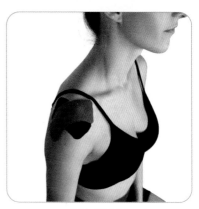

IMAGE 4.14

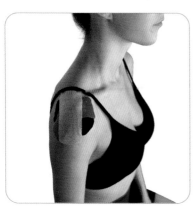

IMAGE 4.15

K-TAPING OF THE SHOULDER: BICEPS

▸ **Tape:** 50 mm k-tape.

▸ **Position:** Arm in neutral position with the elbow extended.

▸ **Actions:** To help fluid dynamics to the biceps.

▸ **Indications:** Biceps strain.

▶ **Instructions:** Cut a single length of tape directly down the centre of the tape leaving approximately 7–8 cm for the anchor. Place the anchor over the lower portion of the belly of the biceps. With one leg of the tape, place a 50–75% stretch to the middle portion of the tape, and stretch up and over the area of the long head of biceps. If you have cut the tape a little too long, don't worry and continue the same line of the tape over the shoulder. Repeat with the other leg, but this time over the short head aiming towards the coracoid process. Again, if the tape has been cut a little long, just continue up and over the shoulder (Image 4.16).

▶ **Tip:** This technique is particularly beneficial for chronic bicep tendinopathy.

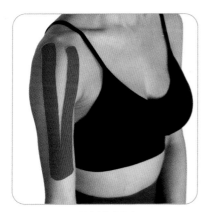

IMAGE 4.16

BIOMECHANICAL TAPING OF THE SHOULDER: INTERNAL ROTATION (COCKING PHASE)

▶ **Tape:** 50 mm or 75 mm biomechanical tape.

▶ **Position:** Shoulder internally rotated (hand on hip).

▶ **Actions:** To support the anterior shoulder, especially for those who play throwing sports or who do overhead work; decelerate external rotation; preload movement into internal rotation; support the gleno-humeral joint by approximating the joint and support the upper limb.

▸ **Indications:** Issues in the cocking phase of throwing; discomfort when working overhead; late stage of rehabilitation of glenohumeral dislocation and instability; weakness in the internal rotators of the glenohumeral joint; pectoral muscle tear or strain.

▸ **Instructions:** Start with a board anchor on the lateral side of the upper arm, under the distal deltoid attachment point (Image 4.17). The tape wraps over the mid to low portion of the biceps (no stretch) angling up as you spiral the tape around the medial side of the arm. Continue up and around the triceps, bringing the tape over and around the anterior portion of the shoulder and across onto the chest.

Make sure that the attachment is fully over the chest – over to the contralateral side is best as short anchors can cause traction blisters (Image 4.18).

▸ **Tip:** This technique can either be used with a laminated strip of bio-mechanical tape or applied twice with tape overlapping.

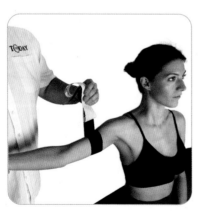
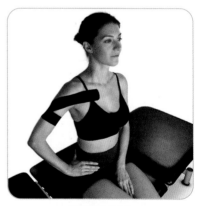

IMAGE 4.17   IMAGE 4.18

BIOMECHANICAL TAPING OF THE SHOULDER: EXTERNAL ROTATION (THROWING PHASE)

▸ **Tape:** 50 mm or 75 mm biomechanical tape.

▸ **Position:** Shoulder externally rotated.

▸ **Actions:** Support the posterior shoulder, and the shoulder at the end of the throwing phase; preload movement into external rotation; support the glenohumeral joint by approximating the joint and support the upper limb.

▸ **Indications:** To support the late stage of rehabilitation of glenohumeral dislocation and instability, weakness in the internal rotators of glenohumeral joint, and pectoral muscle tear or strain.

▸ **Instructions:** Start with a broad anchor on the lateral side of the upper arm, under the distal deltoid attachment point (Image 4.19). The tape wraps over the mid to low portion of the biceps (no stretch), angling up as you spiral the tape around the medial side of the arm (Image 4.20). Continue up and around the triceps, bringing the tape over and around the anterior portion of the shoulder and across onto the back.

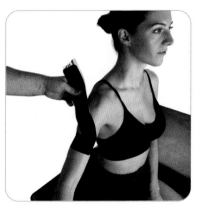

IMAGE 4.19

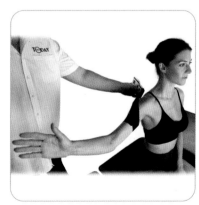

IMAGE 4.20

Make sure that the attachment is fully over the back – over to the contralateral side is best as short anchors can cause traction blisters (Image 4.21).

▶ **Tip:** This technique can either be used with a laminated strip of bio-mechanical tape or applied twice with tape overlapping.

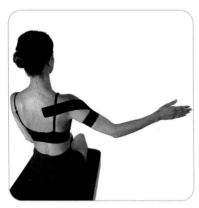

IMAGE 4.21

BIOMECHANICAL TAPING OF THE SHOULDER: BICEPS/SUPRASPINATUS

▶ **Tape:** 50 mm biomechanical tape.

▶ **Position:** Arm in a neutral position.

▶ **Actions:** To help deload biceps and supraspinatus.

▶ **Indications:** Biceps tendinopathy; supraspinatus tendinopathy.

▶ **Instructions:** Cut two lengths of biomechanical tape, one should be slighter longer than the other. Starting with the arm in a neutral position, use the shorter piece of tape and place a long anchor on the lateral side of the upper arm below the deltoid (Image 4.22). Ask your patient to abduct the arm and whilst taking the slack out of the tape, apply it over the deltoid and the tip of the shoulder. Continue along the top of the shoulder over the area of supraspinatus and apply the anchor to the skin. If you have cut the tape a little long, do not continue up the neck but along the base of the neck towards the opposite shoulder (Image 4.23).

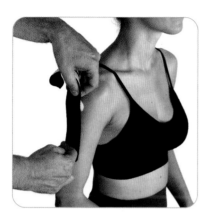

IMAGE 4.22

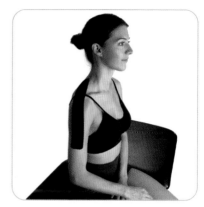

IMAGE 4.23

Ask your patient to supinate their hand palm up. Taking the second strip, place a long anchor over the lower portion of the biceps belly. Ask your patient to flex their shoulder and lift their arm. Whilst taking the slack out of the tape, apply it over the biceps towards the acromioclavicular joint and continue over the shoulder and along the scapula (Image 4.24). If you have cut the tape a little long, continue the line across the back (Image 4.25).

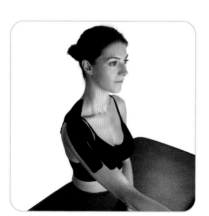

IMAGE 4.24

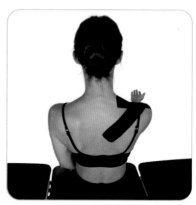

IMAGE 4.25

▸ **Tip:** These techniques are more about the position of the arm whilst taping to create the tension in the tape rather than stretching the tape. Stretching the tape can cause skin traction blisters.

When negotiating around bras and clothing, keep the backing paper on the tape and take off a small part at a time, allowing you to tuck the tape under clothing without getting the tape stuck together.

References

Anderson, M.J., Mack, C.D., Herzog, M.M. and Levine, W.N., 2021. Epidemiology of shoulder instability in the National Football League. *Orthopaedic Journal of Sports Medicine, 9*(5), 23259671211007743.

Cools, A.M., Maenhout, A.G., Vanderstukken, F., Declève, P., Johansson, F.R. and Borms, D., 2021. The challenge of the sporting shoulder: from injury prevention through sport-specific rehabilitation toward return to play. *Annals of Physical and Rehabilitation Medicine, 64*(4), 101384.

Deng, P., Zhao, Z., Zhang, S., Xiao, T. and Li, Y., 2021. Effect of kinesio taping on hemiplegic shoulder pain: a systematic review and meta-analysis of randomized controlled trials. *Clinical Rehabilitation, 35*(3), 317–331.

Dewir, I.M., Ibrahim, A.A., Khaled, O.A. and Hussein, H.M., 2023. Effect of rigid taping versus scapular stabilizing exercises for subacromial impingement syndrome: a randomized triple-blinded controlled trial. *Health, Sport, Rehabilitation, 2025,* 11, 3.

Ghozy, S., Dung, N.M., Morra, M.E., Morsy, S., Elsayed, G.G., Tran, L., Abbas, A.S., Loc, T.T.H., Hieu, T.H., Dung, T.C. and Huy, N.T., 2020. Efficacy of kinesio taping in treatment of shoulder pain and disability: a systematic review and meta-analysis of randomised controlled trials. *Physiotherapy, 107*, 176–188.

Göktaş, H.E., Çitaker, S. and Yurtsever, E.D., 2022. Acute effects of dynamic taping on pain, range of motion and proprioception in patients with subacromial impingement syndrome. *Int J Acad Med Pharm, 4*(2), 35–41.

Hodgetts, C.J., Leboeuf-Yde, C., Beynon, A. and Walker, B.F., 2021. Shoulder pain prevalence by age and within occupational groups: a systematic review. *Archives of Physiotherapy, 11*, 1–12.

Huang, H.M., Hsu, C.Y., Hsieh, I.F., Yang, P.C. and Cheng, Y.H., 2023. The effect of dynamic tape's directional support on shoulder fatigue and pitching performance in amateur baseball players: a randomized crossover trial. *Research Square.* doi:10.21203/rs.3.rs-3593810/v1.

Kim, T., Park, J.M., Kim, Y.H., Park, J.C. and Choi, H., 2022. The short-term effectiveness of scapular focused taping on scapular movement in tennis players with shoulder pain: a within-subject comparison. *Medicine, 101*(39), e30896.

Kraan, R.B., de Nobel, D., Eygendaal, D., Daams, J.G., Kuijer, P.P.F. and Maas, M., 2019. Incidence, prevalence, and risk factors for elbow and shoulder overuse injuries in youth athletes: a systematic review. *Translational Sports Medicine*, 2(4), 186-195.

Letafatkar, A., Rabiei, P., Kazempour, S. and Alaei-Parapari, S., 2021. Comparing the effects of no intervention with therapeutic exercise, and exercise with additional kinesio tape in patients with shoulder impingement syndrome. A three-arm randomized controlled trial. *Clinical Rehabilitation*, 35(4), 558-567.

McConnell, J., Donnelly, C., Hamner, S., Dunne, J. and Besier, T., 2012. Passive and dynamic shoulder rotation range in uninjured and previously injured overhead throwing athletes and the effect of shoulder taping. *PM&R*, 4(2), 111-116.

Olsen, B. and Gregory, B., 2023. Diagnosis and nonoperative treatment of acromioclavicular joint injuries in athletes and guide for return to play. *Clinics in Sports Medicine*, 42(4), 573-587.

Ozer, S.T., Karabay, D. and Yesilyaprak, S.S., 2018. Taping to improve scapular dyskinesis, scapular upward rotation, and pectoralis minor length in overhead athletes. *Journal of Athletic Training*, 53(11), 1063-1070.

Park, S.J. and Kim, S.Y., 2018. The effect of scapular dynamic taping on pain, disability, upper body posture and range of motion in the postoperative shoulder. *Korean Society of Physical Medicine*, 13(4), 149-162.

Park, S.Y., Kim, M.J., Seol, S.E., Hwang, C., Hong, J.S., Kim, H. and Shin, W.S., 2020. Effects of dynamic taping on shoulder joint proprioception. *Physical Therapy Rehabilitation Science*, 9(4), 269-274.

Partner, R., Jones, B., Tee, J. and Francis, P., 2022. Playing through the pain: the prevalence of perceived shoulder dysfunction in uninjured rugby players using the Rugby Shoulder Score. *Physical Therapy in Sport*, 54, 53-57.

Saracoglu, I., Emuk, Y. and Taspinar, F., 2018. Does taping in addition to physiotherapy improve the outcomes in subacromial impingement syndrome? A systematic review. *Physiotherapy Theory and Practice*, 34(4), 251-263.

Schwab, L.M., 2020. Incidence, mechanisms and risk factors for shoulder injuries in community Australian football players (PhD thesis). doi:10.25904/1912/3990.

Snodgrass, S.J., Farrell, S.F., Tsao, H., Osmotherly, P.G., Rivett, D.A., Chipchase, L.S. and Schabrun, S.M., 2018. Shoulder taping and neuromuscular control. *Journal of Athletic Training*, 53(4), 395-403.

Tan, B., Jia, G., Song, Y. and Jiang, W., 2022. Effect of kinesiotaping on pain relief and upper limb function in stroke survivors: a systematic review and meta-analysis. *American Journal of Translational Research*, 14(5), 3372.

Thalagala Arachchige, L.K.N.T. and Parami Irushara Sankalpani, H.A., 2023. Effects of kinesio taping on adhesive capsulitis (Bachelor's thesis).

Tudini, F., Levine, D., Healy, M., Jordon, M. and Chui, K., 2023. Evaluating the effects of two different kinesiology taping techniques on shoulder pain and function in patients with hypermobile Ehlers-Danlos syndrome. *Frontiers in Pain Research*, 4, 1089748.

Turgut, E., Can, E.N., Demir, C. and Maenhout, A., 2023. Evidence for taping in overhead athlete shoulders: a systematic review. *Research in Sports Medicine*, 31(4), 368-397.

Wang, Y., Li, X., Sun, C. and Xu, R., 2022. Effectiveness of kinesiology taping on the functions of upper limbs in patients with stroke: a meta-analysis of randomized trial. *Neurological Sciences*, 43(7), 4145-4156.

Yang, L., Yang, J. and He, C., 2018. The effect of kinesiology taping on the hemiplegic shoulder pain: a randomized controlled trial. *Journal of Healthcare Engineering*, *2018*, 8346432.

4

CHAPTER 5

Elbow

Research evidence

Sports that involve throwing, or using equipment to hit a ball or object, have a high incidence of elbow injuries. The most prevalent are lateral epicondylitis (tennis elbow) and medial epicondylitis (golfer's elbow), common overuse injuries in sport (Fakhre et al., 2020; Li et al., 2019; Meunier, 2020; Hodge, 2023). Sayampanathan et al. (2020) even found that patients who smoked had a higher incidence of lateral epicondylitis. Medial and lateral epicondylitis can also occur in the work environment, especially from manual jobs involving repetitive movements (Bretschneider et al., 2022; Seidel et al., 2019).

Rigid taping of the elbow can be widely seen in contact sports such as rugby, where it can help prevent excessive hyperextension of the elbow when tackling. Taping can also help prevent hyperextension in patients with hypermobility (Callahan et al., 2022). Using rigid taping has also been shown to give short-term pain relief and add pain-free muscle function for lateral epicondylitis (Lucado et al., 2022). Du et al. (2021) found that supporting and restricting excessive movement with rigid tape post-surgery rehabilitation following a terrible triad injury of the elbow produced faster and more efficient improvement in quality of life, pain and range of movement compared to using an external fixation brace.

In the 2021 study by Erpala et al., the application of k-tape was found to have a beneficial effect on lateral epicondylitis after four weeks compared with rest and medication. Due to the effects of k-tape on fluid dynamics, Lee et al. (2020) found that the combination of deep friction massage and taping was beneficial in decreasing pain, improving function and increasing strength in patients with lateral epicondylitis compared to massage alone.

In further studies investigating k-taping for lateral epicondylitis, Shaheen et al. (2019) reported that k-tape was move effective than ultrasound, and Özmen et al. (2021) found that ultrasound, shockwave therapy and k-tape all had a beneficial effect. Therefore, it is clear that using a combination of modalities can increase the therapeutic benefits for patients and their symptoms. This is further supported by studies that found k-taping had only a short-term effect on tendinopathies, therefore illustrating the importance of supplementing taping with loading, stretching and rehabilitation to gain long-term benefits (Ortega-Castillo et al., 2021; Triyanita and Hendrik, 2022).

Hill et al. (2020) observed a decrease in muscle activity in extensor carpi ulnaris and extensor digitorum when using biomechanical taping, illustrating a deloading effect throughout submaximal gripping. This had a beneficial effect on lateral elbow tendinopathy. Deloading of the wrist extensors was also observed in the study by Huang and Kim (2021), in their analysis of repetitive tasks and daily movements and the application of biomechanical tape. Pavani (2021) found that the use of biomechanical tape helped deload the forearm extensors and aided in the rehabilitation of tennis elbow.

Taping of the elbow is most commonly used to prevent excessive mobility of the joint, or to provide support. Evidence also shows that k-tape can benefit patients with lateral epicondylitis (tennis elbow).

Techniques

RIGID TAPING OF THE ELBOW

▸ **Tape:** 38 mm rigid sports tape.

▸ **Position:** Elbow in a semi-flexed position, depending on the level of restriction you require.

▸ **Actions:** To prevent hyperextension of the elbow.

▸ **Indications:** Hyperextension injuries.

▸ **Instructions:** Place two anchors around the arm, one above the elbow approximately one-third along the upper arm and the second below the elbow approximately halfway down the forearm. Both anchors should wrap completely around the arm and forearm respectively (Image 5.1).

Now decide how much extension you need to restrict and ask your patient to hold this position. Starting from the upper anchor, place a strip diagonally across the elbow to the lower anchor on the opposite side and smooth down onto the anchor – note that the middle portion should not be stuck down on the anterior elbow. Repeat this from the upper anchor towards the lower anchor but from the opposite side, creating a cross in front of the elbow (Image 5.2). This process is repeated 2–3 times depending on the level of restriction desired (Image 5.3), making sure that there is always a gap between the skin and the crossing of the tapes.

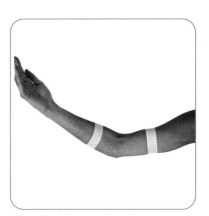

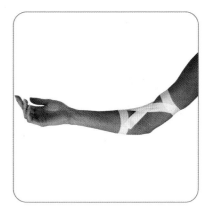

IMAGE 5.1   IMAGE 5.2

After you have achieved the required level of restriction, place a central strip of tape running vertically from the upper to lower anchor (Image 5.4). Once this is done, place a strip of tape around the crossed section of the tapes to prevent the tapes sticking to the anterior elbow. To finish, cover and secure the anchors (Image 5.5). To prevent the tape being pulled off whilst playing sports, it is advisable to either cover with an elasticated sleeve or to wrap with an elastic wrap.

▸ **Tip:** Do not apply the anchors too tightly around the arm, as this will become uncomfortable for your patient.

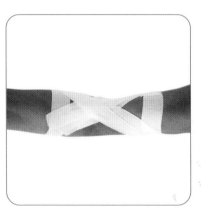

IMAGE 5.3

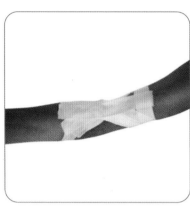

IMAGE 5.4

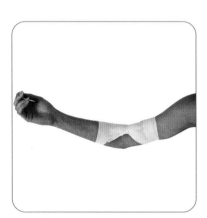

IMAGE 5.5

K-TAPING OF THE ELBOW: LATERAL EPICONDYLITIS

▸ **Tape:** 50 mm k-tape.

▸ **Position:** Elbow in a neutral position.

▸ **Actions:** To support and increase fluid dynamics in the extensor muscles of the forearm.

▸ **Indications:** Lateral epicondylitis (tennis elbow).

▸ **Instructions:** This can be applied in two ways, either with a straight strip or Y-strip (as shown in Image 5.6). The proximal anchor is applied over and just above the lateral epicondyle. With an approximately 50% stretch on the tape, apply over the common extensor tendon and extensor forearm muscles and then apply the anchor with no stretch. If using a Y-strip, apply the anchor as above, then the first leg along the side of the extensor tendon with a 50% stretch, and then apply the anchor. Run the second leg of the tape on the opposite side of the tendon with an approximately 1 cm gap between to the two legs, and apply in exactly the same way (Image 5.6).

To create a false origin along the extensor tendon, apply a strip of k-tape across the first strip at a right angle to the lower tape, approximately one-quarter to one-third of the way along the tape (Image 5.7).

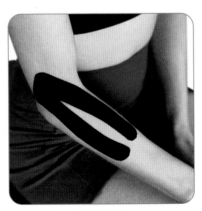
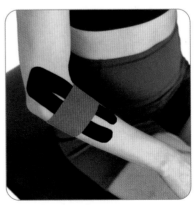

IMAGE 5.6   IMAGE 5.7

▶ **Tip:** With the second strip, palpate along the extensor tendon and feel for a tender trigger point. Once found, apply the second strip directly over this trigger point for extra support.

K-TAPING OF THE ELBOW: MEDIAL EPICONDYLITIS

▶ **Tape:** 50 mm k-tape.

▶ **Position:** Elbow in a neutral position.

▶ **Actions:** To support and increase fluid dynamics in the flexor muscles of the forearm.

▶ **Indications:** Medial epicondylitis (golfer's elbow).

▶ **Instructions:** This can be applied in two ways, either with a straight strip or Y-strip (as shown in Image 5.6). The proximal anchor is applied over, and just above, the medial epicondyle. With an approximately 50% stretch on the tape, apply over the common flexor tendon and flexor muscles of the forearm and then apply the anchor with no stretch. If using a Y-strip, apply the anchor as above, then the first leg along the side of the flexor tendon with a 50% stretch, and then apply the anchor. Run the second leg of the tape on the opposite side of the tendon with an approximately 1 cm gap between the two legs, and apply in the same way.

   To create a false origin along the flexor tendon, apply a strip of k-tape across the first strip at a right angle to the lower tape, approximately one-quarter to one-third of the way along the tape.

▶ **Tip:** With the second strip, palpate along the flexor tendon and feel for a tender trigger point. Once found, apply the second strip directly over this trigger point for extra support.

BIOMECHANICAL TAPING OF THE ELBOW: DELOADING LATERAL EPICONDYLITIS

▸ **Tape:** 50 mm biomechanical tape.

▸ **Position:** Elbow in semi-flexed position and wrist extended (dorsiflexed).

▸ **Actions:** To deload the extensor muscles of the forearm.

▸ **Indications:** Lateral epicondylitis (tennis elbow).

▸ **Instructions:** Once you have measured the length of tape that you require, cut two diamond-shaped holes approximately 5–8 cm from the distal end of the tape (Image 5.8). (You can just tape the dorsal side of the hand, but this method will help the tape last longer, and give more support to any movement).

Place the index and middle fingers through the respective holes and apply the distal anchor onto the palm (Image 5.9). Applying the tape with the wrist in a dorsiflexed position, take the slack out of the tape with a gentle tension and apply the tape onto the forearm. Do not try to stick the tape down to the back of the hand at this point. The proximal anchor runs over and around the lateral epicondyle, and if cut too long, around the upper arm (Image 5.10).

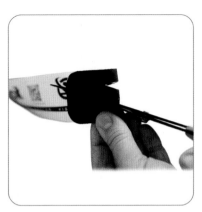

IMAGE 5.8

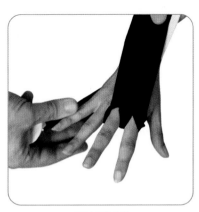

IMAGE 5.9

At this stage bring the palm back to a neutral position and smooth the tape onto the back of the hand and forearm (Image 5.11). For extra support, you can also laminate the tape.

A strip can also be placed over the wrist and mid-forearm to prevent the tape lifting and to give extra support (Image 5.12).

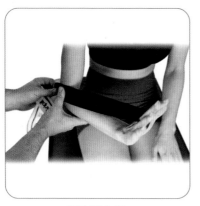

IMAGE 5.10

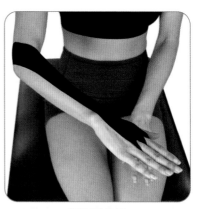

IMAGE 5.11

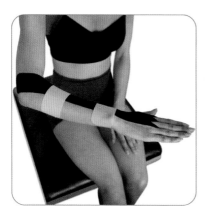

IMAGE 5.12

BIOMECHANICAL TAPING OF THE ELBOW:
DELOADING MEDIAL EPICONDYLITIS

▸ **Tape:** 50 mm biomechanical tape.

▸ **Position:** Elbow in semi-flexed position and wrist flexed (palmar flexed).

▸ **Actions:** To deload the flexor muscles of the forearm.

▸ **Indications:** Medial epicondylitis (golfer's elbow).

▸ **Instructions:** Once you have measured the length of tape that you require, cut two diamond-shaped holes approximately 5–8 cm from the distal end of the tape (Images 5.13 and 5.14). (You can just tape the palm side of the hand, but this method will help the tape last longer, and give more support to the movement).

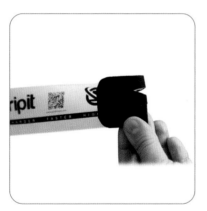
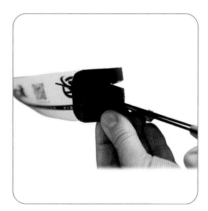

IMAGE 5.13   IMAGE 5.14

Place the index and middle fingers through the respective holes and apply the distal anchor onto the back of the hand (Image 5.15). Applying the tape with the wrist in a palmar-flexed position, take the slack out of the tape with a gentle tension and apply the tape onto the forearm. Do not try to stick the tape down to the back of the hand at this point (Image 5.16). The proximal anchor runs over and around the medial epicondyle, and if cut too long, around the upper arm.

At this stage, bring the hand/wrist back to a neutral position and smooth the tape onto the palm and forearm. For extra support you can also laminate the tape (Images 5.17 and 5.18).

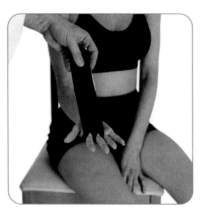

IMAGE 5.15

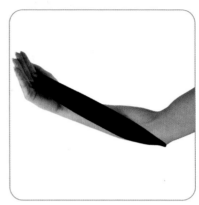

IMAGE 5.16

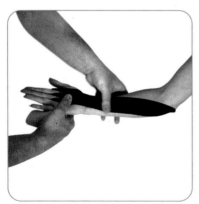

IMAGE 5.17

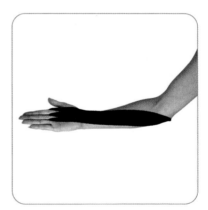

IMAGE 5.18

Strips can also be placed over the wrist and mid-forearm to prevent the tape lifting and to give extra support (Image 5.19).

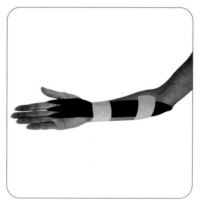

IMAGE 5.19

5

References

Bretschneider, S.F., Los, F.S., Eygendaal, D., Kuijer, P.P.F. and van der Molen, H.F., 2022. Work-relatedness of lateral epicondylitis: systematic review including meta-analysis and GRADE work-relatedness of lateral epicondylitis. *American Journal of Industrial Medicine, 65*(1), 41–50.

Callahan, A., Squires, A. and Greenspan, S., 2022. Management of Hypermobility in Aesthetic Performing Artists: A Review. *Orthopaedic Physical Therapy Practice, 34*(3), 134–145.

Du, S., Wei, L., He, B., Fang, Z., Zhou, E., Ma, X. and Li, J., 2021. Dynamic fixation using rigid tape in rehabilitation after surgery of terrible triad injury of the elbow: a randomized trial. *Journal of Back and Musculoskeletal Rehabilitation, 34*(6), 957–964.

Erpala, F., Ozturk, T., Zengin, E.C. and Bakir, U., 2021. Early results of kinesio taping and steroid injections in elbow lateral epicondylitis: a randomized, controlled study. *Medicina, 57*(4), 306.

Fakhre, E., Means Jr, K.R., Kessler, M.W., Desale, S., Paryavi, E. and Lincoln, A.E., 2020. The epidemiology of hand-to-elbow injuries in United States collegiate sports over 10 academic years. *Athletic Training & Sports Health Care, 12*(4), 159–166.

Hill, C.E., Stanton, R., Heales, L.J. and Kean, C.O., 2020. Therapeutic tape use for lateral elbow tendinopathy: a survey of Australian healthcare practitioners. *Musculoskeletal Science and Practice, 48*, 102160.

Hodge, L.J., 2023. Shoulder and elbow injuries in professional baseball pitchers (PhD dissertation).

Huang, T.Z. and Kim, S.Y., 2021. Effect of forearm dynamic taping on muscle activity of extensor carpi radialis brevis during wrist isometric and isotonic contraction. *Physical Therapy Korea, 28*(2), 93–100.

Lee, J.H., Oh, J.S. and Kim, M.H., 2020. Effect of deep friction massage with taping technique on strength, pain, function and wrist extensor muscle activity in patient with tennis elbow. *Journal of Musculoskeletal Science and Technology*, 4(2), 76–83.

Li, N.Y., Goodman, A.D., Lemme, N.J. and Owens, B.D., 2019. Epidemiology of elbow ulnar collateral ligament injuries in throwing versus contact athletes of the National Collegiate Athletic Association: analysis of the 2009–2010 to 2013–2014 seasons. *Orthopaedic Journal of Sports Medicine, 7*(4), 2325967119836428.

Lucado, A.M., Day, J.M., Vincent, J.I., MacDermid, J.C., Fedorczyk, J., Grewal, R., Martin, R.L., Dewitt, J., Paulseth, S., Dauber, J.A. and Szekeres, M., 2022. Lateral elbow pain and muscle function impairments: clinical practice guidelines linked to the International Classification of Functioning, Disability and Health from the Academy of Hand and Upper Extremity Physical Therapy and the Academy of Orthopaedic Physical Therapy of the American Physical Therapy Association. *Journal of Orthopaedic & Sports Physical Therapy*, 52(12), CPG1-CPG111.

Meunier, M., 2020. Lateral epicondylitis/extensor tendon injury. *Clinics in Sports Medicine, 39*(3), 657–660.

Ortega-Castillo, M., Martin-Soto, L. and Medina-Porqueres, I., 2020. Benefits of kinesiology tape on tendinopathies: a systematic review. *Montenegrin Journal of Sports Science & Medicine, 9*(2), 73–86.

Özmen, T., Koparal, S.S., Karataş, Ö., Eser, F., Özkurt, B. and Gafuroğlu, T.Ü., 2021. Comparison of the clinical and sonographic effects of ultrasound therapy, extracorporeal shock wave therapy, and kinesio taping in lateral epicondylitis. *Turkish Journal of Medical Sciences, 51*(1), 76–83.

Pavani, K. I., 2021. Analyzing the effectiveness of dynamic taping using conventional management in tennis elbow. *Indian Journal of Research in Pharmacy and Biotechnology, 1*(9), 1–22.

Sayampanathan, A.A., Basha, M. and Mitra, A.K., 2020. Risk factors of lateral epicondylitis: a meta-analysis. *The Surgeon, 18*(2), 122–128.

Seidel, D.H., Ditchen, D.M., Hoehne-Hückstädt, U.M., Rieger, M.A. and Steinhilber, B., 2019. Quantitative measures of physical risk factors associated with work-related musculoskeletal disorders of the elbow: a systematic review. *International Journal of Environmental Research and Public Health, 16*(1), 130.

Shaheen, H., Alarab, A. and Ahmad, M.S., 2019. Effectiveness of therapeutic ultrasound and kinesio tape in treatment of tennis elbow. *Journal of Novel Physiotherapy and Rehabilitation*, 3(1), 025–033.

Triyanita, M. and Hendrik, H., 2022. Combination of tapping with eccentric exercise and passive stretching on handgrip ability of elbow tennis patients. *Health Notions, 6*(6), 269–273.

CHAPTER 6

Wrist and Hand

Research evidence

Injuries to the hand are common in sports such as rugby, American football and Australian rules football, where grasp is used both in handling the ball and gripping opponents, and in any sport involving a moving ball, such as basketball, netball, handball, and volleyball. One in four of all fractures involve the wrist and hand. Hand injuries are also commonly seen in baseball, cricket or where there is contact such as ice hockey or hockey.

Hand injuries are equally common in manual handling settings, especially where repetitive tasks are involved (Hayton et al., 2019; Asai et al., 2020; Goes et al., 2020). Conditions such as carpal tunnel syndrome have a higher incidence in people who are obese, do work- or sport-related repetitive wrist tasks, are pregnant, and in conditions such as rheumatoid inflammation (Genova et al., 2020; Battista et al., 2021).

When someone is returning to play or activity after injury, the risk of reinjuring is high. Although rehabilitation guidelines vary from sport to sport, Allahabadi et al. found in their systemic review (2023) that rigid taping of the thumb following ulnar collateral ligament surgery aided rehabilitation and gave athletes reassurance when returning to play. Singh (2019) states that rigid taping is recommended to help stabilize and limit range of movement and is beneficial for sportspersons and athletic performance.

The use of k-tape pre- and post-surgery for carpal tunnel syndrome can be beneficial for patients, and can help with pain relief, whilst also reducing symptoms and scar tissue (Daroglou et al., 2021). Other studies have reported that using k-tape for the treatment of carpal tunnel syndrome helped decrease pain and symptoms, and increased quality of sleep (Kösehasanoğulları et al., 2020; Movaghar et al., 2023).

Aminian-Far et al. (2022) found that k-tape was an effective and conservative treatment choice for carpal tunnel syndrome in manual labourers; compared with wrist splints, k-tape did not restrict daily activities, nor did it produce any side effects.

According to Ortega-Castillo et al. (2020), k-tape gave short-term benefits in the treatment of tendinopathies including De Quervain's tenosynovitis, but further research is needed to establish long-term benefits. Oruk et al. (2023) discovered that using k-tape on the flexor carpi ulnaris, and extensor carpi brevis and longus in darts players improved wrist kinematics and functional performance.

Due to the deloading property of biomechanical tape, it would make sense that biomechanical taping would be beneficial in the management of conditions such as De Quervain's tenosynovitis, but to the date, no research has been carried out apart from case studies. From personal experience, I have found biomechanical taping offers an effective complementary treatment in the management of conditions such as De Quervain's tenosynovitis.

Techniques

RIGID TAPING FOR THUMB SUPPORT

▸ **Tape:** 38 mm rigid tape.

▸ **Position:** Thumb in an extended position, the wrist in a neutral position.

▸ **Actions:** To restrict excessive mobility and prevent further injury of the thumb.

▸ **Indications:** To stabilize the metacarpal and phalangeal joint, and metacarpal and carpal joints.

▸ **Instructions:** An anchor can be applied around the wrist initially if desired. Secure the tape on the dorsal side of the forearm approximately three-quarters of the way down, in a diagonal direction towards the palmar side of the thumb, run the tape without tension (Image 6.1) and wrap around the thumb.

As you come around to the dorsal side of the thumb, continue the angle of the tape diagonally along the thumb towards the wrist on the palmar side (Image 6.2). Continue down across the wrist and wrap around the wrist, with no tension. Repeat with another layer of tape over the first, with a 25–50% overlay.

This is repeated 2–3 times depending on the level of restriction required. Once completed, add an additional anchor around the ends of the tape to tidy up (Image 6.3).

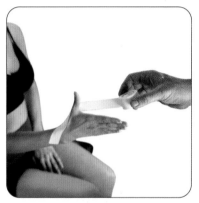

IMAGE 6.1

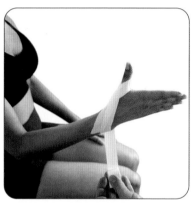

IMAGE 6.2

6

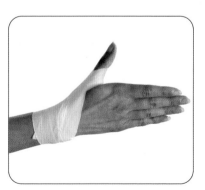

IMAGE 6.3

> ▶ **Tip:** We have not included an initial anchor around the wrist, as it can be too compressive for the wrist. Also, when wrapping around the wrist, make sure there is not too much tension on the tape to avoid causing too much compression and subsequent discomfort.

K-TAPING FOR CARPAL TUNNEL SYNDROME

▶ **Tape:** 50 mm k-tape.

▶ **Position:** Wrist in an extended position.

▶ **Actions:** To lift the tissues over the carpal retinaculum.

▶ **Indications:** Carpal tunnel syndrome.

▶ **Instructions:** Cut two strips of k-tape: the first is a longer strip that will run along two-thirds/three-quarters of the forearm, the second is to wrap around the wrist. Cut the longer strip down the middle, approximately a quarter of the way down the length from both ends. Apply the central anchor with a small amount of stretch, one-quarter to one-third down the length of the forearm from the elbow on the anterior side (Image 6.4).

With a 50% stretch on the tape and the patient's wrist extended, apply one leg of the tape over the forearm and wrist, attaching the anchor over the base of the hand. Repeat the same process with the opposite leg of the tape, and come over the wrist and base of the thumb. Smooth the tape down with no stretch on the anchors. Repeat again with the proximal legs of the tape as shown in Image 6.5.

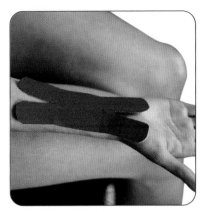

IMAGE 6.4

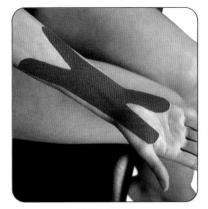

IMAGE 6.5

BIOMECHANICAL TAPING FOR CARPAL TUNNEL SYNDROME

▶ **Tape:** 50 mm biomechanical tape.

▶ **Position:** Hand in a neutral position.

▶ **Actions:** To reduce compression on the carpal tunnel.

▶ **Indications:** Carpal tunnel syndrome.

▶ **Instructions:** Cut a strip of biomechanical tape to a length that will wrap three-quarters of the way around the wrist. Cut a small diamond shape in the tape, approximately 2–4 cm from the end (Image 6.6). Insert this over the thumb and stick it down so that the tape runs over and along the dorsal side of the hand. Add an approximately 50% stretch to the tape, slightly pulling the thumb to open the palmar side of the wrist (Image 6.7). Wrap the tape around the wrist, attaching the anchor to the ulnar side of the wrist (Image 6.8).

▶ **Tip:** Due to washing hands, always apply a pre-tape spray to the area to help adhesion.

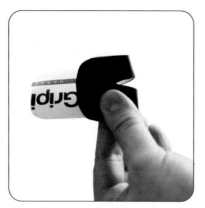

IMAGE 6.6

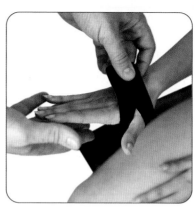

IMAGE 6.7

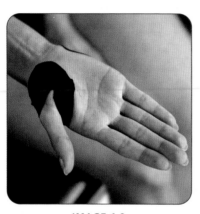

IMAGE 6.8

BIOMECHANICAL TAPING FOR DE QUERVAIN'S TENOSYNOVITIS

▸ **Tape:** 50 mm biomechanical tape.

▸ **Position:** Hand in neutral position.

▸ **Actions:** To unload abductor pollicis longus (APL) and extensor pollicis brevis (EPB).

▸ **Indications:** De Quervain's tenosynovitis.

▸ **Instructions:** Place an anchor strip around the end of the thumb on the dorsal side (nail side). Ask your patient to extend the thumb and slightly abduct the wrist. Take the slack out of the tape by stretching proximally up the forearm and attach the proximal anchor with no stretch on the forearm, approximately halfway along (Image 6.9). The middle part of the tape should not be stuck down at this point.

Once the two anchors are firmly attached, ask the patient to bring the wrist back into a neutral position and palmar flex the thumb. This will bring the middle portion of the tape down onto the skin. Smooth the tape down in this position (Image 6.10).

A small strip can also be placed around the wrist to prevent the tape from lifting (Image 6.11).

▸ **Tip:** To help adhesion to the skin, a small strip of 25 mm rigid tape can be wrapped around the thumb to keep the biomechanical tape in place on the thumb.

6

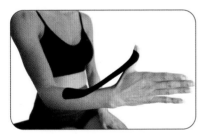

IMAGE 6.9

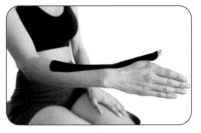

IMAGE 6.10

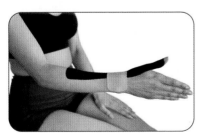

IMAGE 6.11

References

Allahabadi, S., Kwong, J.W., Pandya, N.K., Shin, S.S., Immerman, I. and Lee, N.H., 2023. Return to play after thumb ulnar collateral ligament injuries managed surgically in athletes: a systematic review. *Journal of Hand Surgery Global Online, 5*(3), 349–357.

Aminian-Far, A., Pahlevan, D. and Kohnegi, F.M., 2022. Kinesio taping as an alternative treatment for manual laborers with carpal tunnel syndrome: a double-blind randomized clinical trial. *Journal of Back and Musculoskeletal Rehabilitation, 35*(2), 439–447.

Asai, K., Nakase, J., Shimozaki, K., Toyooka, K., Kitaoka, K. and Tsuchiya, H., 2020. Incidence of injury in young handball players during national competition: a 6-year survey. *Journal of Orthopaedic Science, 25*(4), 677–681.

Battista, E.B., Yedulla, N.R., Koolmees, D.S., Montgomery, Z.A., Ravi, K. and Day, C.S., 2021. Manufacturing workers have a higher incidence of carpal tunnel syndrome. *Journal of Occupational and Environmental Medicine, 63*(3), e120-e126.

Daroglou, S., Lytras, D., Kottaras, A., Iakovidis, P., Kottaras, I. and Chasapis, G., 2021. A review of the efficacy of kinesio taping in carpal tunnel syndrome. *International Journal of Orthopaedics, 7*(2), 513–516.

Genova, A., Dix, O., Saefan, A., Thakur, M. and Hassan, A., 2020. Carpal tunnel syndrome: a review of literature. *Cureus, 12*(3).

Goes, R.A., Lopes, L.R., Cossich, V.R.A., de Miranda, V.A.R., Coelho, O.N., do Carmo Bastos, R., Domenis, L.A.M., Guimarães, J.A.M., Grangeiro-Neto, J.A. and Perini, J.A., 2020. Musculoskeletal injuries in athletes from five modalities: a cross-sectional study. *BMC Musculoskeletal Disorders, 21*, 1–9.

Hayton, M., Ng, C.Y., Funk, L., Watts, A. and Walton, M. eds., 2019. *Sports Injuries of the Hand and Wrist.* Springer International Publishing.

Kösehasanoğulları, M., Yılmaz, N., Karakoyun, A., Şenyuva, İ. and Kösehasanoğulları, S.G., 2020. Investigation of the efficacy of kinesiological banding in pregnancy-related carpal tunnel syndrome. *Selcuk Medical Journal, 36*(2), 109–115.

Movaghar, S., Roostayi, M.M., Naimi, S.S., Daryabor, A., Akbari, N.J. and Mehreganfar, B., 2023. Comparison of 4 weeks of cupping and kinesio-taping on clinical and ultrasound outcomes of carpal tunnel syndrome during pregnancy. *Journal of Bodywork and Movement Therapies, 35*, 57–63.

Ortega-Castillo, M., Martin-Soto, L. and Medina-Porqueres, I., 2020. Benefits of kinesiology tape on tendinopathies: a systematic review. *Montenegrin Journal of Sports Science & Medicine, 9*(2), 73–86.

Oruk, D.Ö., Karakaya, M.G., Yenişehir, S. and Karakaya, İ.Ç., 2023. Effect of kinesio taping on wrist kinematics and functional performance: a randomized controlled trial. *Journal of Hand Therapy, 36*(1), 3–12.

Singh, G., 2019. Athletic taping and its implications in sports. *International Journal on Integrated Education, 2*(4), 1–7.

CHAPTER 7

Hip

Research evidence

Hip pain can mean different things to different people. Classic hip joint pain is felt in the groin over the anatomical location of the hip, however many patients presenting with hip pain will point to their buttocks, which could indicate low back pain referral, gluteal muscle strain, sciatic nerve involvement or hamstring tendinopathy, or to their side, which may raise suspicion of greater trochanteric bursitis, gluteus medius pain or iliotibial band issues. Therefore, when someone presents with 'hip pain', ascertain exactly where the pain is located (Chamberlain, 2021).

Adults over the age of 45 have a 6–10% probability of developing osteoarthritis of the hip, and one in four will develop symptomatic hip osteoarthritis in their lifetime (Fan et al., 2023). Musculoskeletal conditions, are one of the leading causes of pain and disability, and the second largest contributor to years lived with disability, affecting one in five people. Hip pain is the second most common cause of lower limb musculoskeletal pain. (Kemp et al., 2019).

In their 2022 study, Zaworski et al. found that regardless of the type of taping they used (k-tape or rigid tape), a meaningful increase in gluteus medius muscle activation immediately after application was observed.

In the treatment of cane-assisted individuals following a stroke, using a combination of rigid taping and rehabilitation showed improvement in gait stability both immediately and at one month post-intervention (Wang et al., 2022). The research concluded that rigid tape was a useful adjunct to rehabilitation in individuals with chronic stroke.

In their 2022 study of k-taping for iliotibial band syndrome, Watcharakhueankhan et al. report that although only half of the participants benefitted from k-taping, improvements were found in comfort, stability and running performance. Another study investigating k-taping of the hip flexors found that it improved the intermuscular coordination of the lumbo-pelvic-hip complex in healthy patients, and also that myoelectric activity changes in the agonists and synergists in hip extension were produced post-application of k-tape (Kiseljak and Medved, 2023).

By simultaneously taping both the ankle and hip using k-tape in stroke patients, Um et al. (2019) found a favourable effect on gait and balance. Kim and Lee (2020) also found that using k-tape helped in rehabilitation following chronic hemiparesis. Again, this is a great example of how taping combined with manual and rehabilitation therapy complement each other successfully. This can provide the therapist with options for beneficial treatment modalities, and can prove popular with patients who request taping.

In studies of biomechanical tape, Malta et al. (2023) found it had an immediate effect on muscle activation in a group of healthy athletes, Robinson et al. (2019) found that its elastic deloading properties helped reduce symptoms of greater trochanteric pain syndrome and Wu et al. (2022) found that the elastic quality of biomechanical taping benefitted volleyball players in their landing mechanics.

Techniques

K-TAPING OF PIRIFORMIS

▸ **Tape:** 50 mm k-tape.

▸ **Position:** Side-lying with the hip and knee flexed.

▸ **Actions:** To improve fluid dynamics to a muscle injury.

▸ **Indications:** Piriformis pain.

▶ **Instructions:** Cut three lengths of k-tape, with two short pieces of an identical length and one longer strip. With the longer strip, apply the anchor over the edge of the sacrum, and apply the middle portion of the tape with a 25–50% stretch aiming towards the greater trochanter (Image 7.1).

Apply the second strip at approximately 45 degrees to the first strip, and over the middle portion of the tape with an approximately 50–75% stretch (Image 7.2). Repeat with the third strip at a 45 degree angle to the second tape (Image 7.3).

▶ **Note:** The photos have been taken with the tape over the model's clothes for modesty, but within clinic this needs to be placed directly on the skin.

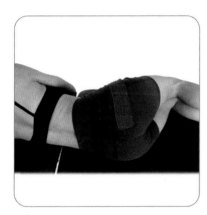

IMAGE 7.1

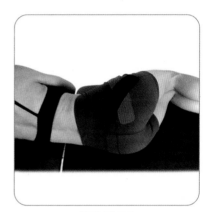

IMAGE 7.2

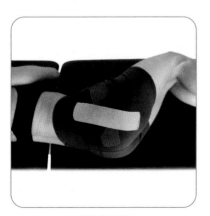

IMAGE 7.3

▶ **Tape:** 75 mm biomechanical tape (laminated).

▶ **Position:** Patient standing in a lunge position with the back leg fully externally rotated, with approximately 40 degrees of abduction and 20 degrees of extension.

▶ **Actions:** To resist hip adduction, flexion and internal rotation.

▶ **Indications:** Valgus at the knees; trochanteric bursitis.

▶ **Instructions:** Starting from the middle of the thigh, apply a large anchor tape with no stretch on the medial side of the thigh (Image 7.4). Wrap around the thigh in a superior lateral direction whilst taking the slack out of the tape. Spiral around the thigh coming over the upper anterior thigh and continue around over the lateral hip (Image 7.5). Cross over the buttock and sacroiliac joint, wrapping around to lie over the anterior superior iliac spine. Apply a large anchor with no stretch (Image 7.6).

   Repeating the process on the opposite leg (Image 7.7) will give support for both hips (Image 7.8), or it can be done with just a single leg.

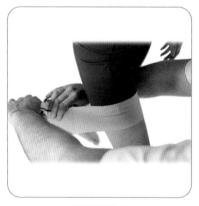

IMAGE 7.4

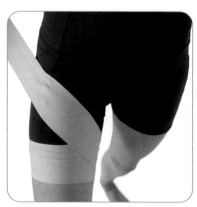

IMAGE 7.5

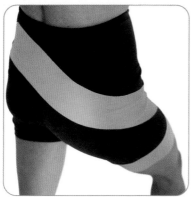

IMAGE 7.6

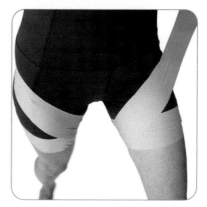

IMAGE 7.7

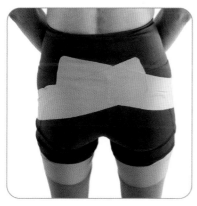

IMAGE 7.8

7

▶ **Note:** The photos have been taken with the tape over the model's clothes for modesty, but within clinic this needs to be placed directly on the skin.

BIOMECHANICAL TAPING FOR DELOADING ILIOPSOAS

▸ **Tape:** 75 mm biomechanical tape (laminated).

▸ **Position:** Hip in slight flexion or neutral.

▸ **Actions:** To deload iliopsoas.

▸ **Indications:** Iliopsoas hypertension.

▸ **Instructions:** Laminate two long strips of biomechanical tape. With a long anchor, lay the superior portion of the tape onto the abdomen, 7–10 cm from the midline, depending on the size of the patient, and 10–15 cm below the rib cage. With little to no stretch on the middle portion of the tape, run the tape inferiorly towards the medial portion of quadriceps (Image 7.9). As you will need to go under the underwear to get skin contact, clearly explain what you will be doing before you proceed, and gain explicit informed consent before applying the tape (see tip).

Apply the distal portion of the tape to the anterior thigh and smooth it down. Make sure you continue to approximately mid-thigh to avoid skin traction and blistering on the thigh (Image 7.10).

▸ **Tip:** Due to the large stresses going through the anchors, make sure you use extra-long anchors.

▸ As an alternative to asking for consent to go under the patient's underwear, simply lay the upper portion of the tape over the abdomen and down towards the underwear. You can explain how the tape needs to be applied to the skin and the direction, and then leave the room to allow the patient to undress or let them adjust the underwear to apply the tape themselves. Once the tape has been applied and the patient is happy for you to re-enter the room, simply check if the tape has been applied correctly. This avoids any embarrassment or awkwardness between you and your patient.

▶ **Note:** The photos have been taken with the tape over the model's clothes for modesty, but within clinic this needs to be placed directly on the skin.

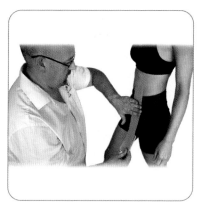
IMAGE 7.9

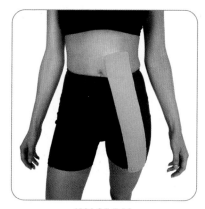
IMAGE 7.10

References

Chamberlain, R., 2021. Hip pain in adults: evaluation and differential diagnosis. *American Family Physician, 103*(2), 81–89.

Fan, Z., Yan, L., Liu, H., Li, X., Fan, K., Liu, Q., Li, J.J. and Wang, B., 2023. The prevalence of hip osteoarthritis: a systematic review and meta-analysis. *Arthritis Research & Therapy, 25*(1), 51.

Kemp, J., Grimaldi, A., Heerey, J., Jones, D., Scholes, M., Lawrenson, P., Coburn, S. and King, M., 2019. Current trends in sport and exercise hip conditions: intra-articular and extra-articular hip pain, with detailed focus on femoroacetabular impingement (FAI) syndrome. *Best Practice & Research Clinical Rheumatology, 33*(1), 66–87.

Kim, K.H. and Lee, Y.J., 2020. Immediate effects of kinesio taping of tibialis anterior and ankle joint on mobility and balance ability for chronic hemiparesis: randomized controlled cross-sectional design. *Physikalische Medizin, Rehabilitationsmedizin, Kurortmedizin, 30*(06), 350–357.

Kiseljak, D., Medved, V., 2023. The effects of Kinesio Taping® on muscle interplay within the lumbo–pelvic–hip complex: a randomized placebo-controlled trial. *Sports, 11*(3), 70.

Malta, V.M., Coelho, A.C., Teruyu, A.I., Silva, G.C., Thomazinho, R.G. and Lobato, D.F., 2023. Immediate effects of Dynamic Tape™ on hip muscle activation and torque and on lower limb kinematics: a randomized controlled clinical trial. *Research in Sports Medicine.* doi:10.1080/15438627.2023.2220060.

7

Robinson, N.A., Spratford, W., Welvaert, M., Gaida, J. and Fearon, A.M., 2019. Does Dynamic Tape change the walking biomechanics of women with greater trochanteric pain syndrome? A blinded randomised controlled crossover trial. *Gait & Posture*, *70*, 275–283.

Um, Y.J., Jang, H.Y. and Lee, S.M., 2019. Taping therapy simultaneously applied to the ankle and hip joint: effect on balance and gait in patients with chronic stroke. *The Journal of Korean Physical Therapy*, *31*(1), 49–55.

Wang, R.Y., Lin, C.Y., Chen, J.L., Lee, C.S., Chen, Y.J. and Yang, Y.R., 2022. Adjunct non-elastic hip taping improves gait stability in cane-assisted individuals with chronic stroke: a randomized controlled trial. *Journal of Clinical Medicine*, *11*(6), 1553.

Watcharakhueankhan, P., Chapman, G.J., Sinsurin, K., Jaysrichai, T. and Richards, J., 2022. The immediate effects of Kinesio Taping on running biomechanics, muscle activity, and perceived changes in comfort, stability and running performance in healthy runners, and the implications to the management of iliotibial band syndrome. *Gait & Posture*, *91*, 179–185.

Wu, C.K., Lin, Y.C., Lai, C.P., Wang, H.P. and Hsieh, T.H., 2022. Dynamic taping improves landing biomechanics in young volleyball athletes. *International Journal of Environmental Research and Public Health*, *19*(20), 13716.

Zaworski, K., Baj-Korpak, J., Kręgiel-Rosiak, A. and Gawlik, K., 2022. Effects of Kinesio Taping and rigid taping on gluteus medius muscle activation in healthy individuals: a randomized controlled study. *International Journal of Environmental Research and Public Health*, *19*(22), 14889.

7

CHAPTER 8

Knee

Research evidence

About 73% of people over the age of 55 have osteoarthritis, with the knee being the most commonly affected joint, followed by the hip (WHO, 2023), and there is a 30% prevalence rate of knee osteoarthritis in former athletes (Madaleno, 2018). So proper treatment and rehabilitation is key for both short- and long-term management of patients presenting with knee pain.

Anatomically, the knee comprises two joints, the patella-femoral and tibio-femoral. Most knee injuries in younger athletes are a result of repetitive and overuse movements, with common injuries including anterior knee pain syndrome, Sinding-Larson-Johanssen syndrome, Osgood-Schlatter disease, and tendonitis around the knee (Patel and Villalobos, 2017). Repetitive movements or prolonged pressure such as from kneeling can result in conditions such as superficial bursitis (housemaid's or carpet fitter's bursitis) (Khodaee, 2017), or retro-patellar bursitis, causing patella-femoral pain.

Pain within the patella-femoral joint is particularly common in young athletes who take part in squatting, cycling and running sports, and in individuals who sit for prolonged periods with their knees flexed at 90 degrees. Shen et al. (2021) found that patella-femoral pain is one of the most frequent presentations in orthopaedic clinics, with patellar maltracking in both adults and adolescents being a common cause.

In their 2023 study, Songur et al. reported that using appropriate taping techniques increased functionality and decreased pain in participants with patella-femoral pain. Balba et al. (2018) found that using rigid sports tape combined with strength training and neuromuscular exercises was an effective treatment combination for medial compartment knee osteoarthritis. During post-recovery from anterior cruciate ligament injury, Huang et al. (2021) found that supporting the knee with protective rigid taping, specifically into knee abduction, internal rotation and extension, had an immediate effect on knee stability and injury prevention, particularly in the landing mechanics of the knee.

A variety of studies have shown that the use of k-tape combined with exercise for the treatment of osteoarthritis in the knee was more effective than exercise alone (Al Khozamy and Al Hamaky, 2023; Mahmoud, 2023; Mohamed and Alatawi, 2023; Lu et al., 2018). Compared with conventional treatment, Mao et al. (2021) found significant effects with k-tape and conventional treatment on isometric muscle strength and pain in patients with osteoarthritis.

Lemos et al. (2023) found that applying k-tape to the rectus femoris increased muscle activity immediately and 24-hours post-application. Kielė and Solianik (2023) studied participants with anterior cruciate ligament tears, and found that k-tape produced short-term improvements in pain and muscle weakness. They also reported that taping combined with rehabilitation gave superior results compared to rehabilitation alone. This is supported in the studies by Lin et al. (2020), Nabil et al. (2021) and Oğuz et al. (2021), which found that taping combined with rehabilitation yielded improved results in pain management compared with exercise alone. In addition, a meta-analysis by Ye et al. (2020) found that using k-tape for osteoarthritic knees significantly improved pain, physical function, range of motion and strength in the quadriceps.

Xiang et al. (2023) report that using k-tape or elastic taping had a role in reducing potential injury to the meniscus and anterior cruciate ligaments in landing phases of the knee, by buffering and decreasing the stress on the knee. Also, with people who had poor control into internal rotation of the knee, elastic taping improved dynamic control thus preventing injury. This is supported in the study by Wu et al. (2022), which found that biomechanical taping of the knee not only helped anterior-posterior joint laxity, but also provided a biomechanical protective effect in the management and prevention of anterior cruciate ligament injuries.

Biomechanical taping can also help reduce the risk of injury during sports and help in improving the valgus angle of the knee in single leg squatting, in research by Ha et al. (2020). Bittencourt et al. (2017) researched the application of biomechanical tape in volleyball players to decrease the frontal plane knee projection angle during single leg squatting. They concluded that the application of biomechanical tape enhances the quality of movement and prevents knee injuries.

Techniques

RIGID TAPING OF THE MEDIAL AND LATERAL KNEE

▸ **Tape:** 38 mm sports tape.

▸ **Position:** Knee in a semi-flexed position.

▸ **Actions:** To support the lateral/medial knee; to stabilize the medial/lateral collateral ligaments.

▸ **Indications:** Support of side and rotational movement of knee; collateral ligament instability.

▸ **Instructions:** Place the first anchor superior to the patella, approximately one-quarter of the way up the thigh. Make sure the tape has no tension placed on it to avoid the tape being too compressive on the thigh, and to allow natural muscle movement. The second anchor wraps around one-quarter to one-third of the way down the calf inferior to the patella. As above, do not place tension on the tape, and wrap completely around the calf (Image 8.1).

From the superior anchor, place a strip diagonally and inferiorly and attach to the lower anchor. Next place a second strip from the superior anchor running diagonally inferior in the opposite direction to the previous strip, forming a cross on the side of the knee (Image 8.2). Continue to repeat the pattern with a 25–50% overlay to the previous tape until you are happy with the coverage and support

(Image 8.3). Extra layers can be applied depending on the level of support required. To finish, place a top anchor completely around the thigh and calf covering all the tape ends and repeat if needed (Image 8.4).

▸ **Tip:** Make sure the anchors are not too compressive around the thigh or calf.

▸ This technique is exactly the same whether applying to the medial or lateral aspect of the knee.

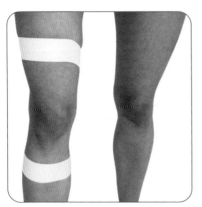

IMAGE 8.1

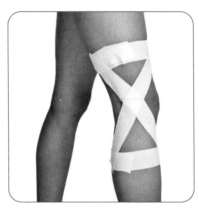

IMAGE 8.2

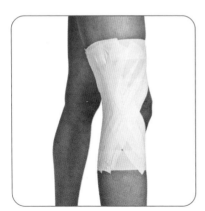

IMAGE 8.3

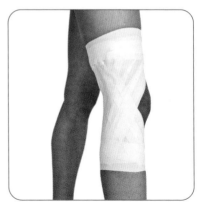

IMAGE 8.4

8

K-TAPING FOR RETRO-PATELLAR INFLAMMATION/MALTRACKING PATELLA

▸ **Tape:** 50 mm k-tape.

▸ **Position:** Knee in 45–90-degree flexion.

▸ **Actions:** To lift tissue around the patella; help with drainage and patella tracking.

▸ **Indications:** Retro-patellar inflammation; maltracking of the patella.

▸ **Instructions:** Cut two strips of 50 mm k-tape, and cut down the centre of each one leaving 7–10 cm at the end for the anchor. The first strip should resemble an upside-down Y. Apply the top anchor of the tape approximately 5 cm above the patella. With an approximately 50% stretch on the tape, place one tail of the tape curving around and over the edge of the patella (the edge of the patella should be around mid-depth of the tape). Continue around the edge of the patella and apply the anchor over the front of the shin (Image 8.5). Repeat the process with the second tail on the opposite side, with the lower anchors crossing over each other on the front of the shin near or over the tibial tuberosity (Image 8.6).

8

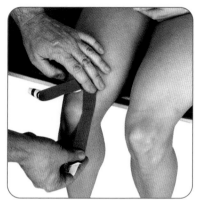
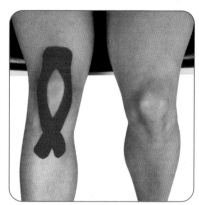

IMAGE 8.5   IMAGE 8.6

This technique is very versatile and can help with lateral or medial maltracking of the patella, or retro-patellar inflammation depending on the placement of the second tape strip.

Placing the second strip so it looks like a Y, apply the anchor over the tibial tuberosity. If you are trying to help with lifting the tissues around the patella for bursitis or retro-patellar inflammation, apply the outer strip over the first strip with a 50% stretch and an approximately 50% overlay, with the top anchor applied over the bottom anchor of the first strip. Repeat the process with the second strip, this time applying over the inner strip with a 50% stretch and 50% overlay again. The anchors should cross over each other on the front of the thigh (Image 8.7). If done correctly the skin over the patella will lift as shown in Image 8.8.

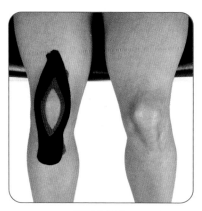

IMAGE 8.7

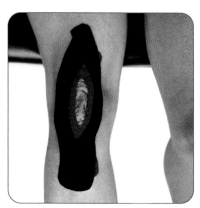

IMAGE 8.8

This technique can also be modified to help maltracking of the patella. For lateral tracking of the patella, instead of applying the outer tape with a 50% overlay on the first tape, apply the outer tail of the second tape directly over the first with a 50% stretch, and then apply the inner tail in exactly the same way as above. This places pressure on the outer border of the patella, thus helping to correct the tracking. For medial tracking of the patella the process is repeated in the opposite way to the above, with the inner tail of the second tape applied directly over the inner tape, and the outer tape is overlaid by 50%, thus placing more pressure over the inner border of the patella.

For tibial tuberosity problems including Osgood-Schlatter's disease, placing a strip horizontally across the patellar ligament with a 50% stretch helps take some pressure off the quadriceps attachment.

▸ **Tip:** Remember, taping on its own will not correct maltracking: to achieve the best results, it should be used in combination with a rehabilitation programme at the same time.

K-TAPING OF THE KNEE FOR HAMSTRING STRAIN

▸ **Tape:** 50 mm/100 mm k-tape (depending on area and size of patient).

▸ **Position:** Knee in extended position.

▸ **Actions:** To support muscle; aid proprioception; increase blood flow to injured muscle.

▸ **Indications:** Muscle (hamstring) strain.

▸ **Instructions:** Start with the patient in the prone position with the knee fully extended. Apply a large anchor to the superior aspect of the thigh, and with an approximately 50% stretch to the middle portion of the tape, smooth the tape along the length of the muscle. With no stretch, apply a large anchor to the opposite end (Image 8.9). Palpate along the muscle where you feel there may be a trauma/tear to the muscle, and apply a short length of k-tape perpendicular to the original strip (Image 8.10). This will cause some restriction and tension to the original length at this section, adding extra support to this area.

▸ **Tip:** Although we have described this technique in the setting of hamstring strains, this principle can be applied to all muscle strains, and using a cross strip will help lift and support any muscle trauma.

8

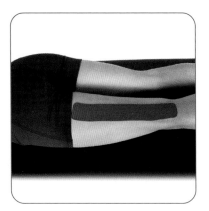

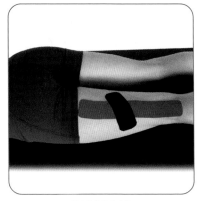

IMAGE 8.9   IMAGE 8.10

BIOMECHANICAL TAPING FOR DELOADING QUADRICEPS/MALTRACKING PATELLA

▶ **Tape:** 75 mm Active Tape (can laminate).

▶ **Position:** Knee in extended position.

▶ **Actions:** To deload the quadriceps muscles; maltracking patella.

▶ **Indications:** Quadriceps strains; maltracking of the patella; deloading in Osgood-Schlatter's disease.

▶ **Instructions:** Cut one strip of 75 mm Active Tape, and cut it down the centre, approximately halfway along. The strip should resemble an upside-down Y. Apply the top anchor of the tape over the anterior surface of the thigh. Whilst taking the slack out of the tape, place one tail of the tape curving around and over the edge of the patella (the edge of the patella should be around the mid-depth of the tape). Continue around the edge of the patella and place the anchor over the front of the shin. Repeat the process with the second tail on the opposite side (Image 8.11), or the anchors can be linked together as shown in Image 8.12. If anchors have been cut too long, continue the line of the tape down and across the lower leg.

Due to the rigidity of k-tape, for rigid support over the patellar ligament apply a strip of 50 mm k-tape horizontally over the patellar ligament; for extra deloading of the patellar ligament, a 50 mm strip of Active Tape can be used in exactly the same way.

▶ **Tip:** Remember, taping on its own will not correct maltracking: to achieve the best results, it should be used in combination with a rehabilitation programme at the same time.

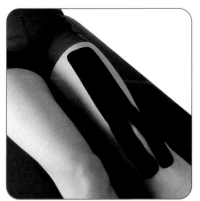
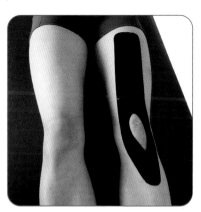

IMAGE 8.11   IMAGE 8.12

8

BIOMECHANICAL TAPING FOR LATERAL COLLATERAL SPRAINS/MENISCAL SUPPORT

▶ **Tape:** 50 mm/75 mm biomechanical tape (can laminate).

▶ **Position:** Knee in semi-flexed position.

▶ **Actions:** To support the lateral collateral ligament; to limit and support internal rotation of the lower leg.

▶ **Indications:** Lateral collateral sprains; meniscal support.

▸ **Instructions:** Starting from the medial side of the lower leg, wrap around the whole of the lower leg and return to the original starting anchor. Add a 25% stretch to the tape and continue diagonally superior from below the patella and over the lateral collateral area (Image 8.13), finishing in the region of the mid-thigh (Image 8.14). If you haven't laminated the tape, repeat the process with a second layer of Active Tape with a 50% overlay on the original tape (Image 8.15).

To fully support the lateral collateral ligament, apply a vertical strip with a 25–50% stretch to the middle of the tape along the medial side of the knee.

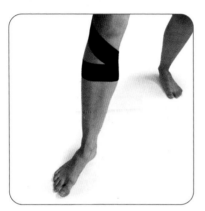

IMAGE 8.13

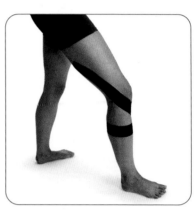

IMAGE 8.14

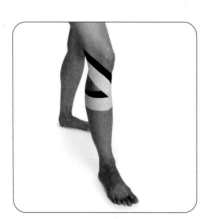

IMAGE 8.15

BIOMECHANICAL TAPING FOR MEDIAL COLLATERAL SPRAINS/MEDIAL MENISCUS TEAR

▸ **Tape:** 50 mm/75 mm biomechanical tape (can laminate).

▸ **Position:** Knee in semi-flexed position.

▸ **Actions:** To support the medial collateral ligament; to limit and support external rotation of the lower leg.

▸ **Indications:** Medial collateral sprains; medial meniscus tear.

▸ **Instructions:** Starting from the lateral side of the lower leg, wrap around the whole of the lower leg and return to the original starting anchor. Add a 25% stretch to the tape and continue diagonally superior from below the patella and over the medial collateral area (Image 8.16), finishing in the region of the mid-thigh. If you haven't laminated the tape, repeat the process with a second layer of Active Tape with a 50% overlay on the original tape (Images 8.17 and 8.18).

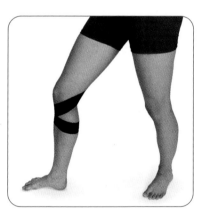

IMAGE 8.16

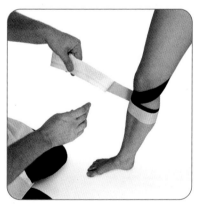

IMAGE 8.17

8

To fully support the medial collateral ligament, apply a vertical strip with a 25–50% stretch to the middle of the tape along the medial side of the knee.

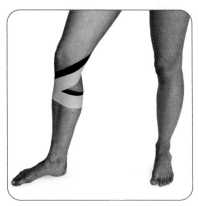

IMAGE 8.18

BIOMECHANICAL TAPING FOR DELOADING HAMSTRINGS

▸ **Tape:** 100 mm biomechanical tape (laminated).

▸ **Position:** Knee in semi-flexed position.

▸ **Actions:** To deload hamstrings.

▸ **Indications:** Hamstring strains.

▸ **Instructions:** Starting with the patient in the prone position with the knee semi-flexed, place a large anchor on the upper portion of the posterior thigh. Do not try to lay the middle of the tape onto the thigh: instead, take the slack out of the middle portion of the tape with a small amount of stretch, and apply the second anchor on the lower leg on the calf (Image 8.19). At this stage the patient allows the leg to extend, and as the knee extends, smooth the middle of the tape along the thigh (Image 8.20). To support the middle portion of the tape and prevent it from lifting, place a horizontal strip across the tape with a 25% stretch at the most (Image 8.21).

▸ **Tip:** Use large, long anchors to prevent skin traction blisters.

8

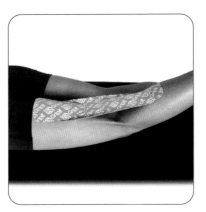

IMAGE 8.19

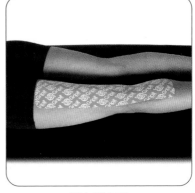

IMAGE 8.20

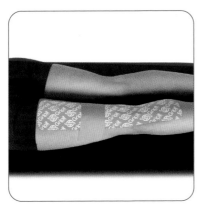

IMAGE 8.21

8

BIOMECHANICAL TAPING FOR DELOADING TIBIALIS ANTERIOR (SHIN SPLINTS).

▸ **Tape:** 50 mm/75 mm biomechanical tape (depending on size of patient).

▸ **Position:** Foot in neutral position.

▸ **Actions:** To support and deload tibialis anterior.

▸ **Indications:** Shin splints.

▸ **Instructions:** With the foot in a neutral position, place a long anchor onto the dorsum (top). As you take the slack out of the tape, ask your patient to dorsiflex their foot, and place a good long top anchor on the front of the shin approximately three-quarters of the way up (Image 8.22). Ask your patient to slowly return the foot to neutral and to point the foot, and as they do this, smooth the tape down onto the shin (Image 8.23).

In most circumstances you will only need one layer, but if you want to create more tension, a second layer can be applied. To secure the tape, place a strip of biomechanical tape across the bottom anchor on the dorsum of the foot and also over the top anchor on the shin. This will help secure the anchors, and also distribute the load on these areas to avoid skin blisters. A third strip can be placed over the mid portion to prevent the tape from lifting (Image 8.24).

▸ **Tip:** Make sure you use good long anchors for this technique to avoid skin drag.

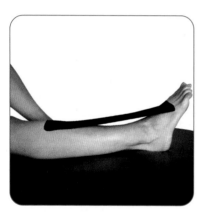

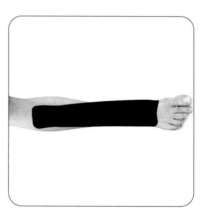

IMAGE 8.22   IMAGE 8.23

▸ K-tape can also be used for this technique (not shown) but with the foot in a plantar flexed starting position. This creates skin lift to increase fluid dynamics to the area, and is useful for acute and chronic

8

presentations. Again, biomechanical tape is used for the support strips, as unlike k-tape, it is stretchy across its width.

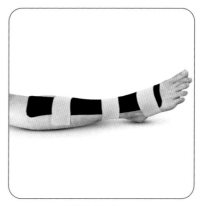

IMAGE 8.24

References

Al Khozamy, H.M. and Al Hamaky, D.M.A., 2023. The influence of combined kinesiotaping and proprioceptive training in knee osteoarthritis. *The Egyptian Journal of Hospital Medicine, 92*, 6858–6862.

Balba, A.E.A., Nada, A.A., Ahmed, H. and Mohammed, M.M., 2018. Effect of neuromuscular training with rigid tape versus strength training on functional performance of knee osteoarthritis. *The Medical Journal of Cairo University, 86*, 241–253.

Bittencourt, N., Leite, M., Zuin, A., Pereira, M., Gonçalves, G. and Signoretti, S., 2017. Dynamic taping and high frontal plane knee projection angle in female volleyball athletes. *British Journal of Sports Medicine, 51*(4), 297–298.

Ha, T.W., Park, S.H. and Lee, M.M., 2020. Comparison of difference in muscle activity ratio, ground reaction force and knee valgus angle during single leg squat and landing according to dynamic taping. *Physical Therapy Rehabilitation Science, 9*(4), 281–286.

Huang, Y.L., Lin, K.W., Chou, L.W. and Chang, E., 2021. Immediate effect of anterior cruciate ligament protective knee taping on knee landing mechanics and muscle activations during side hops. *International Journal of Environmental Research and Public Health, 18*(19), 10110.

Khodaee, M., 2017. Common superficial bursitis. *American Family Physician, 95*(4), 224–231.

Kielė, D. and Solianik, R., 2023. Acute effects of kinesiotaping on pain and muscle strength in individuals with anterior cruciate ligament tear. *Physikalische Medizin, Rehabilitationsmedizin, Kurortmedizin*.

Lemos, T.V., de Souza Junior, J.R., dos Santos, M.G.R., Rosa, M.M.N., Filho, L.G.C. and Matheus, J.P.C., 2023. Kinesio Taping™ effects with different directions and tensions on the muscle activity of the rectus femoris of young adults with a muscle imbalance promoted by mechanical vibration: a randomized controlled trial. *Bulletin of Faculty of Physical Therapy, 28*(1), 33.

8

Lin, C.H., Lee, M., Lu, K.Y., Chang, C.H., Huang, S.S. and Chen, C.M., 2020. Comparative effects of combined physical therapy with kinesio taping and physical therapy in patients with knee osteoarthritis: a systematic review and meta-analysis. *Clinical Rehabilitation, 34*(8), 1014–1027.

Lu, Z., Li, X., Chen, R. and Guo, C., 2018. Kinesio taping improves pain and function in patients with knee osteoarthritis: a meta-analysis of randomized controlled trials. *International Journal of Surgery, 59*, 27–35.

Madaleno, F.O., Santos, B.A., Araújo, V.L., Oliveira, V.C. and Resende, R.A., 2018. Prevalence of knee osteoarthritis in former athletes: a systematic review with meta-analysis. *Brazilian Journal of Physical Therapy, 22*(6), 437–451.

Mahmoud, W.S., 2023. Effect of kinesio taping and exercise on functional impairment in patients with different degrees of knee osteoarthritis. *Isokinetics and Exercise Science*, (preprint), 1–11.

Mao, H.Y., Hu, M.T., Yen, Y.Y., Lan, S.J. and Lee, S.D., 2021. Kinesio taping relieves pain and improves isokinetic not isometric muscle strength in patients with knee osteoarthritis: a systematic review and meta-analysis. *International Journal of Environmental Research and Public Health, 18*(19), 10440.

Mohamed, S.H.P. and Alatawi, S.F., 2023. Effectiveness of kinesio taping and conventional physical therapy in the management of knee osteoarthritis: a randomized clinical trial. *Irish Journal of Medical Science, 192*(5), 2223–2233.

Nabil, M.A.A., Engy, F., Ahmed, F.S. and Abeer, A., 2021. Comparison between effect of McConnell tape, kinesiology tape and open knee brace in treatment of patellofemoral pain. *The Medical Journal of Cairo University, 89*, 1889–1898.

Oğuz, R., Belviranlı, M. and Okudan, N., 2021. Effects of exercise training alone and in combination with kinesio taping on pain, functionality, and biomarkers related to the cartilage metabolism in knee osteoarthritis. *Cartilage, 13*(1_suppl), 1791S-1800S.

Patel, D.R. and Villalobos, A., 2017. Evaluation and management of knee pain in young athletes: overuse injuries of the knee. *Translational Pediatrics, 6*(3), 190.

Shen, A., Boden, B.P., Grant, C., Carlson, V.R., Alter, K.E. and Sheehan, F.T., 2021. Adolescents and adults with patellofemoral pain exhibit distinct patellar maltracking patterns. *Clinical Biomechanics, 90*, 105481.

Songur, A., Demirdel, E., Kılıc, O., Akin, M.E., Alkan, A. and Akkaya, M., 2023. The effects of different taping methods on patellofemoral alignment, pain and function in individuals with patellofemoral pain: a randomized controlled trial. *PM & R: The Journal of Injury, Function, and Rehabilitation.* doi:10.1002/pmrj.13067.

World Health Organisation (WHO), 2023. Osteoarthritis. Accessed March 2024 at: www.who.int/news-room/fact-sheets/detail/osteoarthritis#:~:text=About%20 73%25%20of%20people%20living,and%20the%20hand%20(2).

Wu, C.K., Lin, Y.C., Lai, C.P., Wang, H.P. and Hsieh, T.H., 2022. Dynamic taping improves landing biomechanics in young volleyball athletes. *International Journal of Environmental Research and Public Health, 19*(20), 13716.

Xiang, F., Tang, S., Ou, L., Lin, X. and Chen, J., 2023. Effects of different taping methods on knee joint stress during drop jump landing. *Chinese Journal of Tissue Engineering Research, 27*(30), 4850.

Ye, W., Jia, C., Jiang, J., Liang, Q. and He, C., 2020. Effectiveness of elastic taping in patients with knee osteoarthritis: a systematic review and meta-analysis. *American Journal of Physical Medicine & Rehabilitation, 99*(6), 495–503.

8

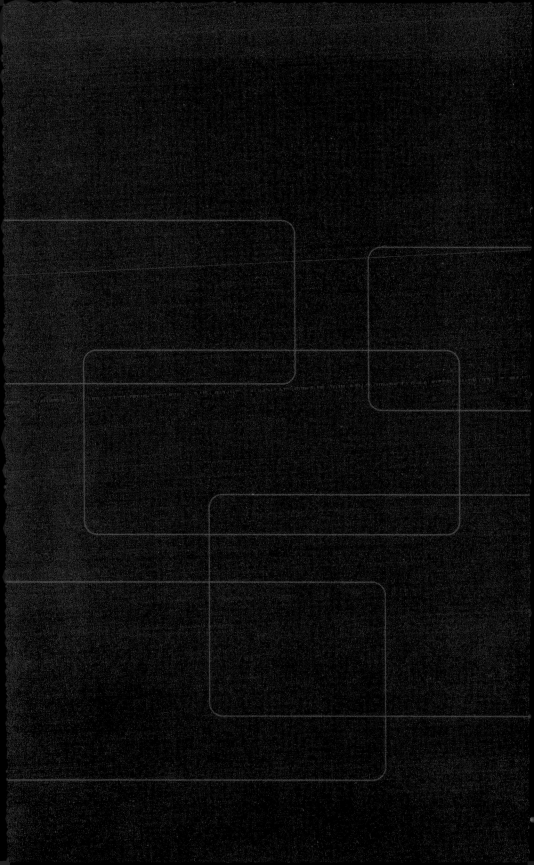

CHAPTER 9

Ankle

Research evidence

Ankle sprains are one of the most common sports injuries you will see in the athlete. Having tools in your repertoire such as taping allows you to provide the best preventative treatment to the individual. Supporting the ankle is often necessary for sports that have high incidences of ankle injuries, such as netball and basketball. Tummala et al. (2023) found that there was a higher incidence of ankle injuries in the National Basketball Association (NBA) compared with other professional sports. Basketball shoes will typically have higher sides to help reduce ankle torsion and may help to reduce the likelihood of sprains. This is also seen in activities such as hiking, where the sides of the boot will often be higher, for the same purpose. Without adequate support, there is a risk of ligament injury from rolling, or spraining an ankle during quick changes of direction.

Studies investigating sports taping of the ankle found that sprain injury rates were reduced (Doshi and Wakode, 2021), with one study reporting a reduction of 50% (Altaweel and Alabbad, 2020). Rigid Achilles tendon taping has a similar effect on gait parameters in overweight and obese individuals: after rigid taping, Shrestha et al. (2023), found there was a significant improvement in stride length, step length and cadence in the study population before and after Achilles taping. From this they hypothesized that rigid taping was effective in preventing excessive joint motion and enhancing proprioception.

Taping in the acute phases following ankle injury can provide compression and protection to the ankle, which may help to reduce inflammation and pain. However, rigid taping must be used with care, as applying too compressive and restrictive taping during the inflammatory stage can also be harmful and lead to increased symptoms and further complications, such as compartment syndrome.

Kaminski et al. (2019) reported that sports taping effectively reduced the risk of lateral ankle sprains in uninjured and previously injured populations. Shumway and Vraa (2022), found that a multimodal approach of rigid sports taping to stabilize ankles and manual therapy was useful in reducing pain and improving function of the ankle. Due to the restriction and support of sports tape, Alawna et al. (2021) found there was a significant improvement in proprioception and balance in uninjured participants. Pratola and Sanzo (2023) also found that rigid taping helped provide ankle stability in basketball players, however the restriction of movement caused by the rigid taping had a negative effect on vertical jumping height. Therefore, it must be understood that although restricting the mobility of the joint will prevent injury, it can have a negative effect on the usage of the joint. As you gain stability, you'll lose mobility, and a balance needs to be found.

A meta-analysis by Biz et al. (2022) showed that k-tape improved gait function and range of movement, and decreased muscle activation. They concluded that the moderate stabilization of k-tape was an effective tool for supporting chronic ankle injuries in athletes. Khalili et al. (2022) showed that the application of k-tape combined with balance training had more of a positive effect than balance exercises alone in improving balance, stability and severity of ankle instability in athletes.

Further studies of k-taping have found that its use in chronic ankle injuries helped improve range of movement in the ankle and improved athletic performance (Sarvestan and Svoboda, 2019); it was effective in reducing calf pain after running and lengthened the time before fatigue affected the calves among athletes (Malhotra et al., 2022), and it had significant benefits in the stability and support of ankle joints in ballet dancers (Botsis et al., 2019). By supporting the Achilles tendon with k-tape, Cheraghi et al. (2022) observed benefits in ankle stability and performance in participants with chronic ankle instability, and Ju (2023) reported that using a combined approach of k-taping the Achilles tendon and treating the plantar fascia eased neuralgic pain in the feet.

Dones et al. (2020) concluded that biomechanical taping was effective when combined with physical therapy and rehabilitation for patients with acute ankle inversion strains, and suggested that the stability achieved with biomechanical taping may underpin the improvement in pain and function with patients. Pawik et al. (2022) observed that dynamic (biomechanical) taping made a significant improvement in balance and coordination in patients with grade I–II ankle sprains. When using biomechanical tape to support plantar flexion of the foot, Song et al. (2022) found that it was effective in increasing the endurance of the calf muscles. Additionally, when biomechanical tape was applied to the calves and Achilles tendon, it was found to enhance balance and control in patients with chronic ankle instability (Kodesh et al., 2021).

Ankle sprains can be serious and cause significant amounts of pain and swelling. After one sprain, the ankle may never regain full stability, leaving it at risk of second or recurrent sprains. This is reflected in research by Desai et al. (2022), which reviewed NFL players over three seasons (2015–2018) and found that ankle injuries hampered players' performance even several years after the initial occurrence, resulting in decreased games played and decrease in performance output per game played. Therefore, if we can prevent injury or enhance recovery by taping, the better the outcome for the athlete.

Techniques

RIGID TAPING FOR ANKLE SUPPORT

▶ **Tape:** 38 mm rigid tape.

▶ **Position:** Foot in a neutral position.

▶ **Actions:** To support the ankle.

▶ **Indications:** Ankle stability.

▶ **Instructions:** Apply an anchor strip around the distal lower leg, just below the belly of the gastrocnemius muscle (Image 9.1).

To prevent inversion sprains, start from the anchor on the medial side of the leg. Lay the tape vertically down over the medial malleolus under the foot and vertically up over the lateral malleolus to the anchor on the lateral side (Image 9.2). Repeat with a second strip with a 50% overlay on the first strip, and for extra support, repeat again with a third strip with a 50% overlay on the second (Image 9.3).

For eversion sprains, start from the lateral side of the anchor, and lay the tape vertically down over the lateral malleolus, under the foot, and up to the anchor of the medial side. Do not place too much tension on the tape as this can prevent expansion of the foot when weight bearing, and become uncomfortable for your patient. Repeat with a second strip with a 50% overlay on the first strip, and for extra support, repeat again with a third strip with a 50% overlay on the second.

For cross-over stirrup support after an inversion sprain, start from the lateral side of the anchor and diagonally cross the tape over the shin towards the medial malleolus. Lay the tape over the plantar side of the foot and over the lateral malleolus, and diagonally cross over the first strip and attach the medial side of the anchor. To prevent excessive eversion in the ankle, repeat the same process as above but start from the medial malleolus and cross over to the lateral malleolus, pass under the foot, and cross over to the lateral anchor. Repeat with a second strip with a 50% overlay on the first strip, and for extra support, repeat again with a third strip with a 50% overlay on the second (Image 9.4).

With no tension on the tape, wrap over the ends of the tape securing the tape down. To tidy everything, repeat with a 50% overlay, repeating down the leg, making sure you do not compress the lower leg (Image 9.5).

▶ **Tip:** To aid tape removal, you can apply underwrap around the lower leg and foot first (Image 9.6). When layering the tape under the foot, try not to layer too heavily over one area, as this can cause discomfort in the foot.

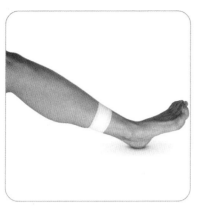

IMAGE 9.1

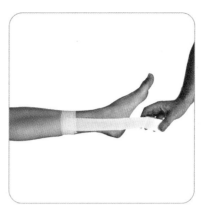

IMAGE 9.2

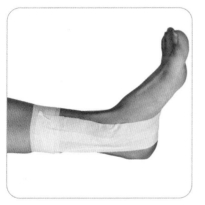

IMAGE 9.3

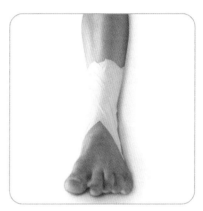

IMAGE 9.4

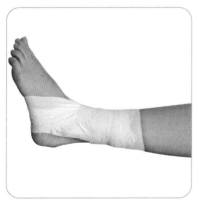

IMAGE 9.5

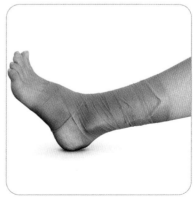

IMAGE 9.6

9

K-TAPING FOR ANKLE SPRAINS

▸ **Tape:** 50 mm k-tape.

▸ **Position:** Foot and ankle in a neutral position.

▸ **Actions:** To improve fluid drainage following ankle sprain.

▸ **Indications:** Post-ankle sprain inflammation and bruising.

▸ **Instructions:** Cut two pieces of 50 mm k-tape directly down the middle, stopping 5–7 cm from the end – these will be the anchors of the tapes. Place the anchor of the first tape on the outside of the lower leg a few centimeters above the swollen or bruised ankle. With an approximately 50–75% stretch, bring one leg of the tape directly down over the bruising or swelling of the lateral ankle, and lay 5 7 inches of end anchor with no stretch. Repeat with the other leg of the k-tape with approximately 1–2 cm between the two legs of the tape (Image 9.7).

Lay the anchor of the second piece of k-tape on the front of the lower leg. Spread the legs of the tape approximately 1–2 cm apart, and with a 50–75 % stretch, apply them over the first layer of tape at an angle. This will produce a criss-cross pattern on the leg over the bruising and swelling, thus aiding fluid dynamics around the ankle (Image 9.8).

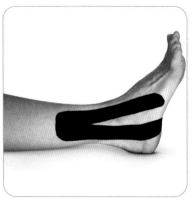

IMAGE 9.7

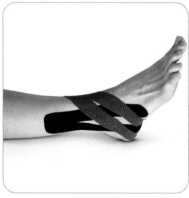

IMAGE 9.8

▸ **Tip:** Due to the constant rubbing of clothes or shoes, using pre-tape spray on the area before applying helps the tape last a little longer.

K-TAPING FOR ACHILLES TENDONITIS

▸ **Tape:** 50 mm k-tape.

▸ **Position:** Patient prone with foot and ankle in neutral position.

▸ **Actions:** To support Achilles tendon; aid proprioception.

▸ **Indications:** Achilles tendonitis; calf strain.

▸ **Instructions:** Cut two lengths of k-tape, and make a long Y-cut in one of them. With the first (unsplit) strip, apply the anchor on the plantar side of the heel, and with an approximately 50% stretch, lay the k-tape over the Achilles tendon and continue up the centre of the calf (Image 9.9). With the second strip, place the distal anchor over the plantar side of the heel covering the first tape, but approximately 2cm beyond the edge of the first so that the second tape is sticking to skin. Lay over the Achilles tendon and the first tape, place an approximately 50% stretch to one leg of the tape and lay over the outer border of the calf. Repeat this on the other side of the calf (Image 9.10).

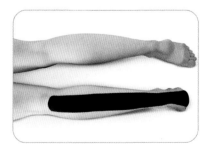
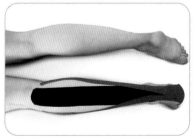

IMAGE 9.9   IMAGE 9.10

BIOMECHANICAL TAPING FOR DELOADING THE ACHILLES TENDON

▶ **Tape:** 50 mm or 75 mm biomechanical tape.

▶ **Position:** Patient prone with ankle in plantar flexed position.

▶ **Actions:** To support the ankle and sub-talar joint; to deload Achilles tendon.

▶ **Indications:** Deloading Achilles tendon following calf strain or Achilles tendonitis.

▶ **Instructions:** Cut two equal lengths of biomechanical tape. Start by placing a long anchor on the lateral side of the heel with the tape running inferiorly and under the heel, then up over the middle and lateral side of the Achilles tendon. Continue superiorly over the lateral belly of the calf (Image 9.11). With the second strip, place the anchor over the medial/plantar side of the heel and lay the tape under the heel and superiorly over the Achilles tendon, crossing the first tape supporting the Achilles tendon. Continue superiorly over the medial belly of the calf (Image 9.12).

▶ **Tip:** Adding more tension to either the medial or lateral side of the heel can help place the heel in a more neutral position. This can help with rehabilitation and also place less strain on the Achilles tendon and help stabilize the ankle joint.

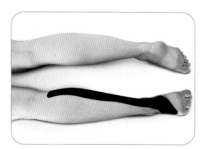

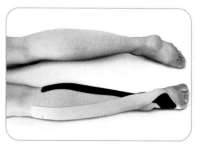

IMAGE 9.11   IMAGE 9.12

BIOMECHANICAL TAPING FOR INVERSION SUPPORT

▸ **Tape:** 50 mm or 75 mm biomechanical tape (can be laminated; if not laminated, will need repeating twice).

▸ **Position:** Initial starting position of the foot and ankle is neutral, but changes through the technique.

▸ **Actions:** To support the ankle, preventing inversion of the foot.

▸ **Indications:** Recovering ankle sprain; 'weak' ankle prone to inversion sprains.

▸ **Instructions:** Place a long anchor on the front of the shin, diagonally angling the tape towards the inside of the foot (Image 9.13). As you bring the tape under the sole of the foot, add a little stretch to the tape and whilst everting the foot, come over the top of the foot angling the tape superiorly across, and up onto the lower shin and around the inside of the leg whilst keeping tension/stretch on the tape (Image 9.14).

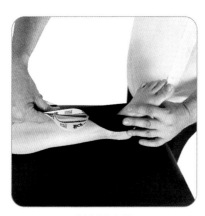

IMAGE 9.13

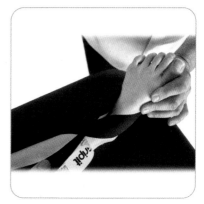

IMAGE 9.14

With no stretch on the tape, wrap the tape around the back of the leg and bring it around the outside of the leg, coming back around towards the original anchor. Continue around again, following a similar direction to the first layer towards the ankle and foot, with a 50% overlay (Image 9.15). Continue to the outside of the foot, everting the foot again, and wrap over the foot towards the inside of the lower leg. If you have cut the tape a little long, continue to wrap around the ankle (Image 9.16).

For full support use a 100 mm biomechanical tape and repeat the first stage of this process, wrapping completely over the first layers of tape (Images 19.17 and 19.18).

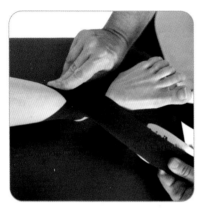

IMAGE 9.15

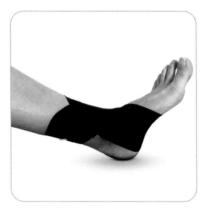

IMAGE 9.16

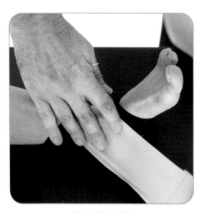

IMAGE 9.17

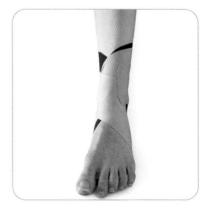

IMAGE 9.18

▶ **Tip:** Do not remove all the backing off the tape, as it will easily get stuck together as you take the tape around the foot. Only take as much backing off the tape as you need.

BIOMECHANICAL TAPING FOR EVERSION SUPPORT/FLAT FEET

▶ **Tape:** 50 mm biomechanical tape.

▶ **Position:** Foot and ankle in a neutral position.

▶ **Actions:** To limit eversion of the ankle.

▶ **Indications:** To help stabilize the ankle into eversion; especially useful for someone who has collapsing aches or needs support.

▶ **Instructions:** Start with an anchor on the medial side of the lower leg a few centimeters above the ankle. In a diagonal and inferior direction and applying a small amount of tension, lay the tape down over the top of the foot and come under the foot. Hold the foot into an inverted position and lay the tape down (Image 9.19). Keeping the foot in an inverted position, bring the tape back over the foot, crossing over the first layer of tape. If you have cut the tape a little too long, continue the tape around the ankle (Image 9.20).

For extra support place another layer around the foot with an approximately 50% overlay (Image 9.21), and for maximum support, another layer of 75 mm tape can be placed over this.

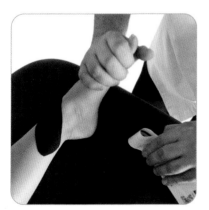

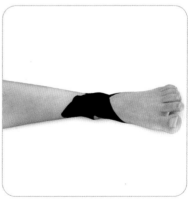

IMAGE 9.19   IMAGE 9.20

9

▶ **Tip:** This technique is more about positioning the foot into inversion when applying the tape to create the tension and support rather than pulling through the tape.

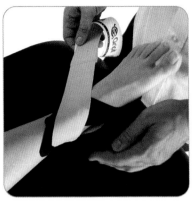

IMAGE 9.21

References

Alawna, M., Unver, B. and Yuksel, E., 2021. Effect of ankle taping and bandaging on balance and proprioception among healthy volunteers. *Sport Sciences for Health, 17*, 665–676.

Altaweel, A. and Alabbad, M.A., 2020. The influence of athletic taping and bracing on ankle sprain: a literature review. *Saudi Journal of Sports Medicine, 20*(2), 36.

Biz, C., Nicoletti, P., Tomasin, M., Bragazzi, N.L., Di Rubbo, G. and Ruggieri, P., 2022. Is kinesio taping effective for sport performance and ankle function of athletes with chronic ankle instability (CAI)? A systematic review and meta-analysis. *Medicina, 58*(5), 620.

Botsis, A.E., Schwarz, N.A., Harper, M.E., Liu, W., Rooney, C.A., Gurchiek, L.R. and Kovaleski, J.E., 2019. Effect of Kinesio® taping on ankle complex motion and stiffness and jump landing time to stabilization in female ballet dancers. *Journal of Functional Morphology and Kinesiology, 4*(2), 19.

Cheraghi, M., Boozari, S., Svoboda, Z., Kovačikova, Z., Needle, A.R. and Sarvestan, J., 2022. Effects of ankle Kinesio™ taping on jump biomechanics in collegiate athletes with chronic ankle instability. *Sport Sciences for Health, 18*(11), 1–8.

Desai, S.S., Dent, C.S., Hodgens, B.H., Rizzo, M.G., Barnhill, S.W., Allegra, P.R., Popkin, C.A. and Aiyer, A.A., 2022. Epidemiology and outcomes of ankle injuries in the National Football League. *Orthopaedic Journal of Sports Medicine, 10*(6), 23259671221101056.

Dones III, V., Tangcuangcoa, L.P., Serraa, M.A., Abada, A., Fuentesa, Z., Josh, P., Labada, J.M.L., Mianoa, J.A.E., Reyesa, G.K., Sabatina, M.R.G. and de Diosa, M.B.V., 2020. Biomechanical taping and standard physical therapy were effective in the management of acute ankle inversion sprain: a pre-and post-intervention study. *Philippine Journal of Allied Health Sciences, 3*(2). doi:10.36413/pjahs.0302.003.

9

Doshi, R. and Wakode, P., 2021. Ankle kinematics after prophylactic ankle taping during sprinting action in recreational players. *International Journal of Physical Education, Sports and Health, 8*(3), 144–147.

Ju, S.B., 2023. Pain reduction effects according to simultaneous application of plantar fascia self-myofascial release therapy and Achilles tendon taping of pedionalgia patients. *Iranian Journal of Public Health, 52*(5), 1095–1096.

Kaminski, T.W., Needle, A.R. and Delahunt, E., 2019. Prevention of lateral ankle sprains. *Journal of Athletic Training, 54*(6), 650–661.

Khalili, S.M., Barati, A.H., Oliveira, R. and Nobari, H., 2022. Effect of combined balance exercises and Kinesio taping on balance, postural stability, and severity of ankle instability in female athletes with functional ankle instability. *Life, 12*(2), 178.

Kodesh, E., Cale'Benzoor, M. and Dar, G., 2021. Effect of dynamic tape on postural sway in individuals with chronic ankle instability. *Journal of Bodywork and Movement Therapies, 28*, 62–67.

Malhotra, D., Sharma, S., Chachra, A., Dhingra, M., Alghadir, A.II., Nuhmani, S., Jaleel, G., Alqhtani, R.S., Alshehri, M.M., Beg, R.A. and Shaphe, M.A., 2022. The time-based effects of kinesio taping on acute-onset muscle soreness and calf muscle extensibility among endurance athletes: a randomized cross-over trial. *Journal of Clinical Medicine, 11*(20), 5996.

Pawik, Ł., Pawik, M., Wysoczańska, E., Schabowska, A., Morasiewicz, P. and Fink-Lwow, F., 2022. In patients with Grade I and II ankle sprains, dynamic taping seems to be helpful during certain tasks, exercises and tests in selected phases of the rehabilitation process: a preliminary report. *International Journal of Environmental Research and Public Health, 19*(9), 5291.

Pratola, M.L. and Sanzo, P., 2023. The effects of ankle taping on measures of ground reaction forces and jump height during a sport-specific vertical jump in youth basketball players. *International Journal of Exercise Science, 16*(6), 898.

Sarvestan, J. and Svoboda, Z., 2019. Acute effect of ankle kinesio and athletic taping on ankle range of motion during various agility tests in athletes with chronic ankle sprain. *Journal of Sport Rehabilitation, 29*(5), 527–532.

Shrestha, A., Goyal, K. and Goyal, M., 2023. Effect of Achilles tendon taping on parameters of gait in asymptomatic overweight and obese individuals. *Revista Pesquisa em Fisioterapia, 13*, e5184-e5184.

Shumway, J.D. and Vraa, D., 2022. Short-term effect of manual therapy & taping on subacute ankle sprains with potential syndesmotic sprain: a case series. *Journal of Manual & Manipulative Therapy, 30*(2), 116–123.

Song, J.Y., Park, S.H. and Lee, M.M., 2022. Comparison of the effects of dynamic taping and kinesio taping on endurance and fatigue of plantar flexor. *Journal of Korean Physical Therapy Science, 29*(1), 73–86.

Tummala, S.V., Morikawa, L., Brinkman, J.C., Crijns, T.J., Vij, N., Gill, V., Kile, T.A., Patel, K. and Chhabra, A., 2023. Characterization of ankle injuries and associated risk factors in the National Basketball Association: minutes per game and usage rate associated with time loss. *Orthopaedic Journal of Sports Medicine, 11*(7), 23259671231184459.

9

CHAPTER 10

Foot

Research evidence

Toe and foot injuries can be common in sports where increased load is put through the foot and toe such as running or climbing, but any sport that places an explosive or repetitive movement through the feet increases the chances of injury (Cobos-Moreno et al., 2022; Almekinders and Engle, 2019). There are higher incidences of foot and toe injuries in males, which could be due to either the type of sports played and/or a higher average body weight loading through the foot (Francis et al., 2019).

Turf toe is a term used for a strain of the hallux (big toe). This is commonly associated with sports that require explosive pushing off through the feet, such as sprinting and American football, especially in running backs, tight ends and wide receivers (Madi et al., 2023). Rigid sports taping has been found to help in the treatment and maintenance of turf toe, due to it decreasing mobility and increasing stability of the hallux (Parekh and Parekh, 2019).

Akaras et al. (2020) found that rigid taping increased the limits of stability and maintained balance in hallux valgus, and Hendley et al. (2021) discovered that using rigid tape in the treatment of turf toe reduced the amount of time taken off from playing.

Rigid sports taping and k-taping can be effective in the support of the lower extremity in running gait, and potentially decrease the risk of developing overuse injuries, as reported by Koens (2019) in their study evaluating the effectiveness of taping in runners.

The use of k-tape for hallux valgus can give short-term relief, and could be an alternative treatment instead of surgery (Żłobiński et al., 2021). The 2021 study by Yu et al. found that k-tape helped improve proprioception of the ankle in inversion during step-down landing stages in both injured and non-injured individuals. Oliveira et al. (2023) also found k-tape effective in helping to aid balance and control in chronic ankle instability.

A common foot problem is plantar fasciitis, affecting the heel of the foot. Taping the foot, or more specifically the plantar fascia, can be very effective. This can create a support or sling for the plantar fascia and so help to take some stress away from it. People who typically suffer with pain are athletes, runners, and other sportspeople. Obesity can also cause significant foot pain and conditions. Taping provides the soft tissues and joints with rest and support to promote healing and recovery.

In their 2022 study, Castro-Méndez et al found that both rigid taping and biomechanical taping had beneficial effects on plantar fasciitis, but that biomechanical taping gave better results in reducing pain intensity. This was reflected by Kim and Lee (2023) in their study comparing k-tape with biomechanical tape, in which they found that biomechanical tape was more effective in regards balance and foot function. The elastic quality of biomechanical tape is possibly the reason why these studies found it to be most effective, which deloads and mimics the function of the plantar fascia.

Techniques

RIGID TAPING FOR TURF TOE

▸ **Tape:** 38 mm rigid tape.

▸ **Position:** Toe in a neutral position.

▸ **Actions:** To limit extension (hyperextension) of the big toe.

▸ **Indications:** Turf toe (metatarsophalangeal joint pain).

▸ **Instructions:** Start by attaching the rigid tape to the plantar side of the big toe (you will not need an initial anchor strip for this technique). Place a small amount of tension on the tape and run towards the heel of the foot along the plantar side of the foot, approximately two-thirds along the plantar surface of the foot (Image 10.1). Depending on how much you want to restrict the toe, you may wish to add a second layer directly over the first (Image 10.2). Once the tape is applied, to help keep it in place wrap a 25 mm strip of tape around the big toe, securing the end of the tape (Image 10.3). Using the 38 mm tape, secure the opposite end by wrapping around the foot (Image 10.4). Make sure not to pull or add tension to the anchor tape, as it will be uncomfortable for the patient if it is too tight.

This technique can also be done with a laminated strip of biomechanical tape: although it will not give as much restrictive support, it will help support the recovering athlete.

▸ **Tip:** Always assess the joint first to determine how much restriction of movement is needed.

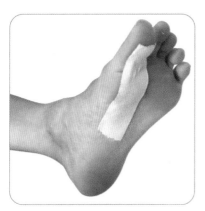

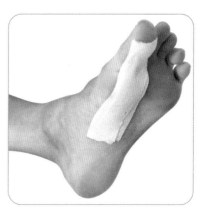

IMAGE 10.1   IMAGE 10.2

10

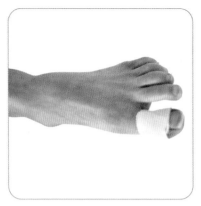
IMAGE 10.3

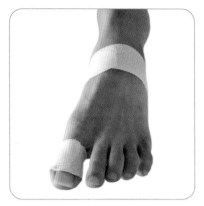
IMAGE 10.4

RIGID TAPING FOR PLANTAR FASCIITIS

▸ **Tape:** 25 mm and 38 mm rigid tape.

▸ **Position:** Foot in a neutral position.

▸ **Actions:** To create a sling to support the plantar fascia.

▸ **Indications:** Plantar fasciitis.

▸ **Instructions:** Using the 25 mm rigid tape, lay an anchor strip from the medial border just proximal to the big toe. Without placing tension on the tape, apply the tape along the medial border of the foot towards the heel (Image 10.5). Wrap around the heel and continue around the lateral border of the foot towards the little toe (Image 10.6).

Next, we need to create a sling to support the plantar fascia: to do this cut a strip of 38 mm tape and attach it on the distal lateral side of the anchor, creating a small squeeze of the foot (make sure you do not squeeze too much as this will cause discomfort when standing on the foot once completed). Attach the tape to the anchor on the opposite side of the foot without pulling or placing tension on the tape (Image 10.7). Now repeat this process with a 50% overlay on the first strip, and continue this process until you reach the heel. You can continue over the heel, but we prefer to leave the heel open as this seems to be more comfortable for patients (Image 10.8).

To help the tape last longer, apply the 25 mm tape without any tension to the distal part of the anchor. Wrap from one side to the opposite side over the top of the foot and attach it to the opposite side. If you wish, you can wrap the tape around the whole foot, but make sure you do not place too much tension on the tape compressing the foot. You can repeat this process over the mid foot (Image 10.9). Once you have completed the transverse sections, place a top anchor over the inner anchor covering the ends of the transverse strips.

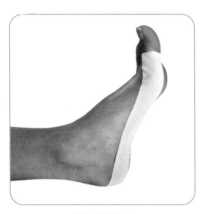

IMAGE 10.5

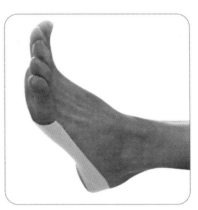

IMAGE 10.6

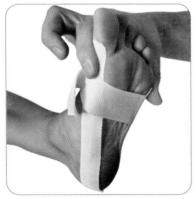

IMAGE 10.7

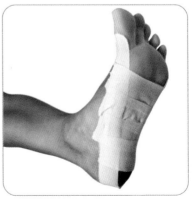

IMAGE 10.8

10

▸ **Tip:** Pinch any folds together and trim, as these can create areas of irritation on the heel and cause discomfort.

You can use 25 mm for all the taping, but using 38 mm tape for the transverse strips saves time and tape.

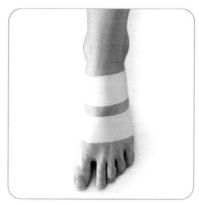

IMAGE 10.9

BIOMECHANICAL/K-TAPING FOR HALLUX VALGUS

▸ **Tape:** 50 mm biomechanical tape/50 mm k-tape.

▸ **Position:** Toe in a neutral position.

▸ **Actions:** To support the big toe and metatarsophalangeal (MTP) joint.

▸ **Indications:** Early hallux valgus (bunion).

▸ **Instructions:** Apply an anchor to the side of the big toe between the big toe and second toe (Image 10.10). Place an approximately 50% tension on the tape (enough to bring the toe back into a neutral or corrected position), and lay the tape along the side of the big toe and along the inside of the foot, approximately halfway along the foot (Image 10.11).

Using another piece of 50 mm tape, apply a 25–50% stretch to the middle of the tape and place over the side of the MTP joint and then along the dorsal and plantar side of the foot with no tension on the anchors (Image 10.12).

For the patient's comfort and to avoid any hotspots, cut off any folds of tape around the toe.

10

▶ **Tip:** This technique can also be used with k-tape but we find that biomechanical tape gives better support.

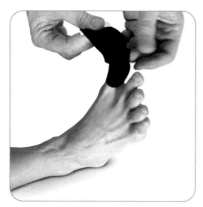

IMAGE 10.10

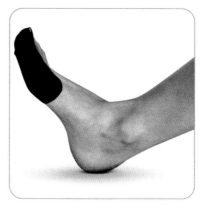

IMAGE 10.11

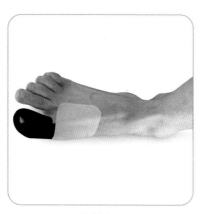

IMAGE 10.12

10

BIOMECHANICAL TAPING FOR
PLANTAR FASCIITIS: TOE WRAP

▸ **Tape:** 75 mm biomechanical tape (laminated).

▸ **Position:** Start with the foot in a neutral position.

▸ **Actions:** To create an elastic sling to support the plantar fascia.

▸ **Indications:** Plantar fasciitis.

▸ **Instructions:** Before placing the tape on the foot, cut three diamond shapes into the tape 7–10 cm from the end of the tape. Slide the diamond holes over the three middle toes, with the short end of the tape wrapped over the dorsal surface of the foot with no stretch (Image 10.13). Ask your patient to gently point their foot. With a small amount of stretch, bring the tape over the heel and stick it down over the back of the heel (Image 10.14). At this time the tape should not be stuck to the plantar surface of the foot. Ask your patient to bring their foot back into a neutral position – this should draw the tape towards the plantar surface. Stick down and smooth the tape to the plantar surface (Image 10.15).

    Cut a second strip of tape and attach the anchor to the dorsal surface of the foot aiming towards the outer/lateral side of the foot. Taking the slack out of the tape, but not placing too much tension on it, wrap under the foot and over the middle portion of the medial arch of the foot (Image 10.16). Continue the line of the tape up onto the leg with a long anchor to prevent traction blistering (Image 10.17).

▸ **Tip:** Pinch any folds around the heel together and trim, as these can create hotspots on the heel and cause discomfort. If the patient is particularly tall or heavy, or will be placing large forces on the foot, you can triple layer the tape along the plantar surface.

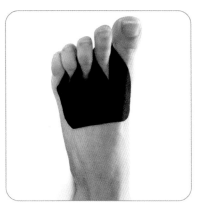

IMAGE 10.13

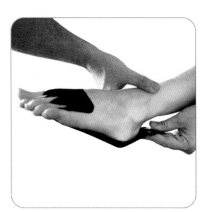

IMAGE 10.14

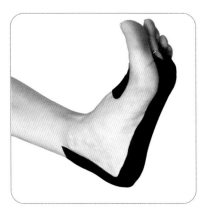

IMAGE 10.15

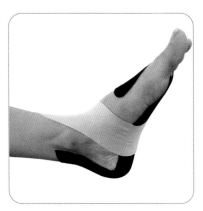

IMAGE 10.16

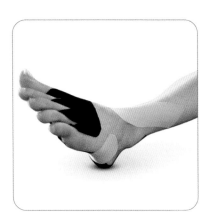

IMAGE 10.17

10

BIOMECHANICAL TAPING FOR PLANTAR FASCIITIS: SLING

▸ **Tape:** 50 mm biomechanical tape (laminated).

▸ **Position:** Start with foot in a neutral position.

▸ **Actions:** To create an elastic sling to support the plantar fascia.

▸ **Indications:** Plantar fasciitis.

▸ **Instructions:** Starting from the big toe, apply the anchor to the plantar side of the toe and wrap around the toe (Image 10.18). With the patient plantar flexing their toe and pointing their foot, take up the tension on the tape, and apply the tape along the medial/inferior portion of the medial arch of the foot (Image 10.19). Wrap the tape around the heel of the foot.

   Once the tape is applied to the lateral side of the heel, come under the foot again with the tape crossing over the first layer, and invert the foot and bring the tape up and over the medial arch. Continue the angle of the tape over the top of the foot onto the lower leg (Image 10.20). If you have cut the tape a little long, continue to wrap around the lower leg with no tension on the tape.

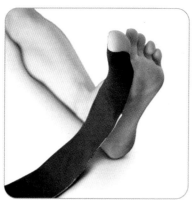

IMAGE 10.18

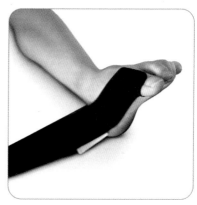

IMAGE 10.19

▶ **Tip:** To prevent the tape coming off the toe, cut and wrap a small piece of tape around the toe. Pinch any folds around the heel together and trim, as these can create hotspots on the heel and cause discomfort.

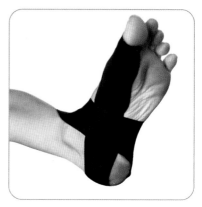

IMAGE 10.20

References

Akaras, E., Guzel, N.A., Kafa, N. and Özdemir, Y.A., 2020. The acute effects of two different rigid taping methods in patients with hallux valgus deformity. *Journal of Back and Musculoskeletal Rehabilitation, 33*(1), 91–98.

Almekinders, L.C. and Engle, C.R., 2019. Common and uncommon injuries in ultra-endurance sports. *Sports Medicine and Arthroscopy Review, 27*(1), 25–30.

Castro-Méndez, A., Palomo-Toucedo, I.C., Pabón-Carrasco, M., Ortiz-Romero, M. and Fernández-Seguín, L.M., 2022. The short-term effect of dynamic tape versus the low-dye taping technique in plantar fasciitis: a randomized clinical trial. *International Journal of Environmental Research and Public Health, 19*(24), 16536.

Cobos-Moreno, P., Astasio-Picado, Á. and Gómez-Martín, B., 2022. Epidemiological study of foot injuries in the practice of sport climbing. *International Journal of Environmental Research and Public Health, 19*(7), 4302.

Francis, P., Whatman, C., Sheerin, K., Hume, P. and Johnson, M.I., 2019. The proportion of lower limb running injuries by gender, anatomical location and specific pathology: a systematic review. *Journal of Sports Science & Medicine, 18*(1), 21.

Hendley, C., May, J., Wallace, J.J. and Cheatham, S.W., 2021. The use of the Mulligan concept for the treatment of a first-degree sprain of the first metatarsophalangeal joint. *Athletic Training & Sports Health Care, 13*(6), e460-e463.

Kim, D.H. and Lee, Y., 2023. Effect of dynamic taping versus kinesiology taping on pain, foot function, balance, and foot pressure in 3 groups of plantar fasciitis patients: a randomized clinical study. *Medical Science Monitor: International Medical Journal of Experimental and Clinical Research, 29*, e941043-1.

10

Koens, N.A., 2019. Evaluating the effectiveness of Kinesio® Tape as an intervention for recreational runners who pronate (PhD thesis, North Dakota State University).

Madi, N.S., Parekh, T.J. and Parekh, S.G., 2023. Outcome of turf toe injuries in NFL players. *The Journal of Foot and Ankle Surgery, 62*(1), 115–119.

Oliveira, G.F.M.D., Stocco, M.R., Macedo, C.D.S.G., Machado, F.V.C., Oliveira, M.R.D. and Andraus, R.A.C., 2023. Different kinesio taping tensions present similar benefits for postural control, dynamic balance, agility and instability sensation in individuals with chronic ankle instability: randomized clinical trial. *Revista Brasileira de Cineantropometria & Desempenho Humano, 25*, e94813.

Parekh, S.G. and Parekh, T.J., 2019. Outcome of turf toe injuries in NFL players. *Foot & Ankle Orthopaedics, 4*(4), 2473011419S00330.

Yu, R., Yang, Z., Witchalls, J., Adams, R., Waddington, G. and Han, J., 2021. Kinesiology tape length and ankle inversion proprioception at step-down landing in individuals with chronic ankle instability. *Journal of Science and Medicine in Sport, 24*(9), 894–899.

Żłobiński, T., Stolecka-Warzecha, A., Hartman-Petrycka, M. and Błońska-Fajfrowska, B., 2021. The short-term effectiveness of kinesiology taping on foot biomechanics in patients with hallux valgus. *Journal of Back and Musculoskeletal Rehabilitation, 34*(4), 715–721.

10

CHAPTER 11

Lymphatic Taping

Research evidence

It is important to reflect on the research regarding k-taping for lymphatic drainage. The theory is that the skin-lifting effect of k-tape creates a space between the top layer of the skin and the underlying tissues, including the fascia. This space induces a pressure gradient between the tissues which allows fluids to move into the lymphatic vessels, resulting in reduced swelling and pain as the healing process is potentially accelerated.

As seen in the images below, instead of using just a strip of tape or a Y-/trouser cut to the tape, a fanning effect is used in order to multiply the lifting effects on the skin and subsequent spacing and pressure gradients within the tissues. The anchor of the tape is placed next to the bruising or oedema, and the legs of the tape are stretched over the area to be treated. There are various ways of doing this, for example by using either straight or waving legs to the tape, and applying two or three layers (we are only showing two layers here but a third can be added). You can also use 50 mm or 100 mm tape depending on the area you are treating. Once you understand the basic principles, you can apply this technique to any area of bruising or swelling, such as taping over oedema from an acute ankle sprain or bruising from a fall.

Cimino et al. (2018) demonstrated that the use of k-tape caused a significant stretch to the epidermis and dermis, thus causing measurable deformities to the skin surface and within the dermis and epidermis, providing plausible pathways in regards the benefits and effects of k-tape on fluid dynamics.

Although Sobiech et al. (2022) found that k-tape did not have an immediate effect on range of movement post-surgery, they did find that k-tape had a positive influence on the absorption of subcutaneous oedema after knee replacement surgery. Labianca et al. (2021) also observed that using k-tape during early rehabilitation after anterior cruciate ligament reconstruction improved post-surgery oedema. Balki and Göktas (2019) correspondingly found k-tape helpful with postsurgical oedema following anterior cruciate reconstruction. Sobiech et al. (2022) likewise found this following primary endoprosthesis of the knee. Hörmann et al. (2020) also found evidence for postoperative oedema efficacy for k-tape.

The study by Baltaci et al. (2023) showed that using k-tape helped to reduce pain and decrease oedema post-surgery. This is also reflected in a meta-analysis by Wang et al. (2024), that found k-tape helped to improve hamstring strength and reduce pain following anterior cruciate ligament reconstruction.

Further research evidence demonstrates that k-taping helps reduce postoperative oedema. The studies by Kasawara et al. (2018), Rostom and El Sayed (2019), Krajczy et al. (2020) and Yilmaz and Ayhan (2023) all report that k-tape has a beneficial effect on inflammation following breast cancer surgery. Lietz-Kijak et al. (2018) also found the same in regards reduction of swelling following orthognathic surgery.

According to a study by Rezaei et al. (2021), the authors observed that although k-taping did not produce a significant change in pain pressure threshold in delayed onset muscle soreness (DOMS) in hamstrings, they did find that it possibly reduced parameters such as pain and range of movement.

Duymaz and Yuksel (2020) concluded in their study that k-taping following acute ankle injuries resulted in reductions in swelling and disability. They also stated that this contributed to faster recovery and healing, which allowed patients to mobilize and rehabilitate quicker.

Therefore the research clearly shows the effectiveness of k-taping in reducing swelling. Early application can help facilitate recovery and rehabilitation.

Technique

K-TAPING FOR LYMPHATIC DRAINAGE

▸ **Tape:** 50 mm or 100 mm k-tape.

▸ **Position:** Area treated in neutral position.

▸ **Actions:** To lift the skin to allow fluid drainage.

▸ **Indications:** Bruising and localized inflammation.

▸ **Instructions:** Depending on the area being treated and size of the patient, use either 50 mm or 100 mm tape (50 mm tape is used in Images 11.1 and 11.2). Cut multiple legs into the tape: a simple way to do this is to first cut centrally along the tape leaving approximately 4 cm for the anchor, and then cut each half into two or three lengths (as in Image 11.1).

Place the anchor next to the area to be treated and smooth down. Place an approximately 50% stretch to one of the central legs of the tape, and either apply it straight as in the images or with a waving line (be as artistic as you want). Smooth it down with a 3–4 cm anchor. Repeat the process with the other central leg of the tape, and continue working from the inner strips outwards – this makes placement of the tape easier (Image 11.1).

If using two strips of k-tape, as shown in Image 11.2, place the anchor of the second strip at an angle to the first and repeat the same procedure. If using three layers this would again be repeated at an angle to the first two patterns.

▸ **Tip:** This technique is shown for the anterior thigh here, but it can be applied to any area of bruising or trauma.

Use a maximum of three strips crossing over, as areas of uncovered skin are required to lift up the skin and fascia to help produce the pressure changes.

11

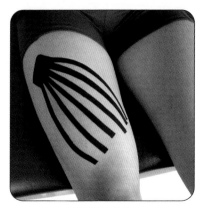

IMAGE 11.1

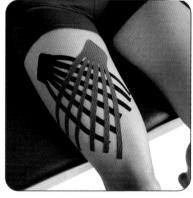

IMAGE 11.2

References

Balki, S. and Göktas, H.E., 2019. Short-term effects of the Kinesio Taping® on early postoperative hip muscle weakness in male patients with hamstring autograft or allograft anterior cruciate ligament reconstruction. *Journal of Sport Rehabilitation, 28*(4), 311–317.

Baltaci, G., Ozunlu Pekyavas, N. and Atay, O.A., 2023. Short-time effect of sterile kinesio tape applied during anterior cruciate ligament reconstruction on edema, pain and range of motion. *Research in Sports Medicine, 31*(5), 550–561.

Cimino, S.R., Beaudette, S.M. and Brown, S.H., 2018. Kinesio taping influences the mechanical behaviour of the skin of the low back: a possible pathway for functionally relevant effects. *Journal of Biomechanics, 67,* 150–156.

Duymaz, T. and Yuksel, S., 2020 Acute treatment of ankle ligament injuries: is kinesio tape effective? *Annals of Clinical and Analytical Medicine.* doi:10.4328/acam.20119

Hörmann, J., Vach, W., Jakob, M., Seghers, S. and Saxer, F., 2020. Kinesiotaping for postoperative oedema – what is the evidence? A systematic review. *BMC Sports Science, Medicine and Rehabilitation, 12*(1), 1–14.

Kasawara, K.T., Mapa, J.M.R., Ferreira, V., Added, M.A.N., Shiwa, S.R., Carvas Jr, N. and Batista, P.A., 2018. Effects of kinesio taping on breast cancer-related lymphedema: a meta-analysis in clinical trials. *Physiotherapy Theory and Practice, 34*(5), 337–345.

Krajczy, M., Krajczy, E., Bogacz, K., Łuniewski, J., Lietz-Kijak, D. and Szczegielniak, J., 2020. The possibility of the use of kinesio taping in internal, oncologic, and neurologic diseases: a systematic review and meta-analysis. *Explore, 16*(1), 44–49.

Labianca, L., Andreozzi, V., Princi, G., Princi, A.A., Calderaro, C., Guzzini, M. and Ferretti, A., 2021. The effectiveness of kinesio taping in improving pain and edema during early rehabilitation after anterior cruciate ligament

11

reconstruction: a prospective, randomized, control study. *Acta Bio Medica: Atenei Parmensis, 92*(6).

Lietz-Kijak, D., Kijak, E., Krajczy, M., Bogacz, K., Łuniewski, J. and Szczegielniak, J., 2018. The impact of the use of kinesio taping method on the reduction of swelling in patients after orthognathic surgery: a pilot study. *Medical Science Monitor: International Medical Journal of Experimental and Clinical Research, 24,* 3736.

Rezaei, M., Mir, S.M., Ghotbi, N., Malmir, K. and Jalaie, S., 2021. Effect of kinesio tape on symptoms induced by delayed onset muscle soreness in hamstrings. *Journal of Modern Rehabilitation, 15*(1), 33–40.

Rostom, E.H. and El Sayed, D.G., 2019. Kineso-taping versus pneumatic compression pump on lymphedema post mastectomy. *Bioscience Research, 16*(2), 1876–1881.

Sobiech, M., Czępińska, A., Zieliński, G., Zawadka, M. and Gawda, P., 2022. Does application of lymphatic drainage with kinesiology taping have any effect on the extent of edema and range of motion in early postoperative recovery following primary endoprosthetics of the knee joint? *Journal of Clinical Medicine, 11*(12), 3456.

Wang, J., Wang, L., Zuo, H., Zheng, C., Wang, G. and Chen, P., 2024. Rehabilitative efficacy of kinesio taping following anterior cruciate ligament reconstruction: a meta-analysis. *Chinese Journal of Tissue Engineering Research, 28*(4), 651.

Yilmaz, S.S. and Ayhan, F.F., 2023. The randomized controlled study of low-level laser therapy, kinesio-taping and manual lymphatic drainage in patients with stage II breast cancer-related lymphedema. *European Journal of Breast Health, 19*(1), 34.

11

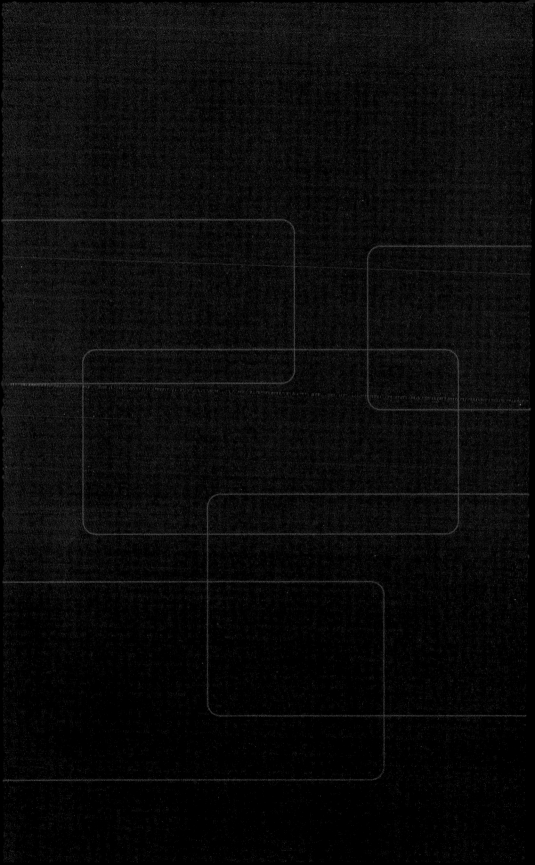

CHAPTER 12

Pregnancy

Research evidence

Many women will experience pelvic girdle and/or low back pain during and after pregnancy (Morino et al., 2024). Taping during pregnancy can be very effective in helping relieve the strain and symptoms associated with the many physiological and mechanical changes the body must go through, and many of the techniques discussed in the other chapters can be beneficial for supporting the low back or thoracic spine. Kesikburun et al. (2018) discuss that musculoskeletal issues and pains can complicate pregnancy more in the third trimester. Bakilan and Zelveci (2020) discuss that early diagnosis and intervention for musculoskeletal problems during pregnancy are vital in their treatment and management.

The research discussed below is focused on the application of taping to the low back. At the time of writing, there aren't any published studies that investigate taping to create a sling for bumps as demonstrated in this chapter. However, anecdotally, I have found this technique to be extremely beneficial for women (including my wife) in relieving the pain and discomfort associated with the lower back and symphysis pubis dysfunction during pregnancy.

In their study of low back pain disability during pregnancy, Aalishahi et al. (2022) found that k-tape not only reduced symptoms immediately, but also provided a lasting effect after it was removed. Xue et al. (2021) found that k-tape application improved low back pain, dysfunction problems and quality of life during pregnancy.

Mohamed and Ikram (2018) found that complementing TENS and paracetamol use with application of k-tape to the low back gave increased benefit to pregnant women compared to TENS and parac-etamol alone. Another study found that elastic taping decreased preg-nancy-related pelvic girdle pain and increased quality of life (Kuciel et al., 2017). Kalinowski and Krawulska (2017) state that k-tape has few side effects during pregnancy, and that the therapeutic effect on low back pain in pregnant women continued after the tape was removed.

In the third trimester, Mutoharoh et al. (2021) observed significant reductions in low back pain when k-tape was combined with maternity exercises, compared with exercise alone. A further study by Kaplan et al. (2016) indicates that k-tape is an effective complementary technique in the treatment of low back pain during pregnancy.

K-tape can also be used post-surgery, as discussed in other chapters. Studies have shown that k-tape reduces post-partum back pain and fatigue, and increases quality of life when applied following caesarean sections (Ali Baraia et al., 2023; Mohamed et al., 2020).

Techniques

The techniques shown in the following images use biomechanical tape due its increased functional support compared to k-tape, but k-tape can be used instead. DO NOT use sports tape for sling techniques as it is too compressive and restrictive to bump and mum.

For these techniques you must use large anchors to avoid skin trac-tion, especially as the skin is already on tension as the bump grows.

BIOMECHANICAL/K-TAPING FOR ABDOMINAL SUPPORT: 1

▸ **Tape:** 75 mm biomechanical tape.

▸ **Position:** Patient in reclined position.

▸ **Actions:** To support bump during pregnancy.

12

▸ **Indications:** Low back pain during pregnancy; symphysis pubis dysfunction.

▸ **Instructions:** Cut two equal lengths of 75 mm biomechanical tape. Starting from one side approximately a quarter of the way around bump from the middle, smooth a very large anchor under the bump going medially and underneath. Ask mum to place one hand over the tape and bump and lift bump as far as comfortable. Whilst taking a little slack out of the tape (DO NOT STRETCH THE TAPE), continue under bump and laterally smooth the tape up whilst coming superiorly and laterally around bump. Place and smooth a very large anchor along the flank of bump and mum. Using the second strip of tape, repeat this process from the opposite side crossing centrally over the first tape, thus giving bump maximum support centrally (Image 12.1).

For extra support, two strips of biomechanical tape can be used either side of the umbilicus. To place these, start with a large anchor inferiorly under bump and ask mum to place one hand over the tape and bump and lift bump. Run the tape directly superiorly over bump and smooth down. Repeat this process on the opposite side (Image 12.2).

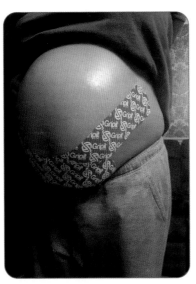

IMAGE 12.1

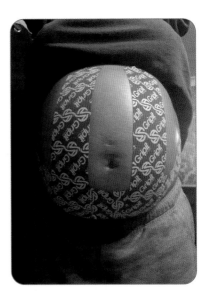

IMAGE 12.2

12

▸ **Tape:** 75 mm biomechanical tape.

▸ **Position:** Patient in reclined position.

▸ **Actions:** To support bump during pregnancy.

▸ **Indications:** Low back pain during pregnancy; symphysis pubis dysfunction.

▸ **Instructions:** First cut two equal lengths of 75 mm biomechanical tape, making sure the tape is long enough to reach around the sides of bump onto the flank of mum. Find the middle of the tape and break the backing of the tape, and using a very large anchor smooth the tape centrally under bump. Ask mum to place one hand over the tape and bump and lift bump as far as comfortable. Whilst taking a little slack out of the tape (DO NOT STRETCH THE TAPE) smooth the tape up and around bump coming superiorly and laterally. Smooth a very large anchor down along the flank. Repeat this process on the other side. For extra support, repeat this process with a second layer of biomechanical tape with an approximately 50% overlay on the first layer (Image 12.3).

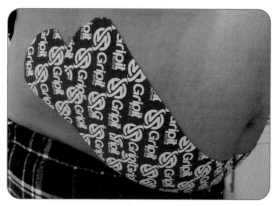

IMAGE 12.3

References

Aalishahi, T., Maryam-Lotfipur-Rafsanjani, S., Ghorashi, Z. and Sayadi, A.R., 2022. The effects of kinesio tape on low back pain and disability in pregnant women. *Iranian Journal of Nursing and Midwifery Research*, 27(1), 41.

Ali Baraia, Z., Ahmed Thabet, H., S Abu Almakarem, A. and Mohamed El-Sayed Atwa, A., 2023. Impact of instructional guidelines regarding kinesio tape on postpartum back pain, fatigue, and disability in women with cesarean section. *Egyptian Journal of Health Care*, 14(4), 479–494.

Bakilan, F. and Zelveci, D.D., 2020. Musculoskeletal problems during pregnancy. *Journal of Clinical Medicine of Kazakhstan*, 6(60), 53–55.

Kalinowski, P. and Krawulska, A., 2017. Kinesio taping vs. placebo in reducing pregnancy-related low back pain: a cross-over study. *Medical Science Monitor: International Medical Journal of Experimental and Clinical Research*, 23, 6114.

Kaplan, Ş., Alpayci, M., Karaman, E., Çetin, O., Özkan, Y., İlter, S., Şah, V. and Şahin, H.G., 2016. Short-term effects of kinesio taping in women with pregnancy-related low back pain: a randomized controlled clinical trial. *Medical Science Monitor: International Medical Journal of Experimental and clinical Research*, 22, 1297.

Kesikburun, S., Güzelküçük, Ü., Fidan, U., Demir, Y., Ergün, A. and Tan, A.K., 2018. Musculoskeletal pain and symptoms in pregnancy: a descriptive study. *Therapeutic Advances in Musculoskeletal Disease*, 10(12), 229–234.

Kuciel, N., Sutkowska, E., Cienska, A., Markowska, D. and Wrzosek, Z., 2017. Impact of kinesio taping application on pregnant women suffering from pregnancy-related pelvic girdle pain – preliminary study. *Ginekologia Polska*, 88(11), 620–625.

Mohamed, H., Yousef, A., Kamel, H.E., Oweda, K. and Abdelsameaa, G., 2020. Kinesio taping and strength recovery of postnatal abdominal muscles after cesarean section. *Egyptian Journal of Physical Therapy*, 4(1), 13–19.

Mohamed, M.Y. and Ikram, I.A., 2018. The influence of application of kinesio taping on pregnancy-related low back pain. *The Medical Journal of Cairo University*, 86(June), 1377–1382.

Morino, S., Ishihara, M., Umezaki, F., Hatanaka, H., Yamashita, M. and Aoyama, T., 2024. History of pain around the lumbopelvic region during perinatal period: a prospective cohort study. *European Spine Journal*, 1–7.

Mutoharoh, S., Astuti, D.P., Kusumastuti, K., Rahmadhani, W. and Phu, P.T., 2021. The effectiveness of pregnancy exercise with kinesio taping on lower back pain in pregnant women in the third trimester. *Jurnal Ilmu Kesehatan Masyarakat*, 12(3), 241–249.

Xue, X., Chen, Y., Mao, X., Tu, H., Yang, X., Deng, Z. and Li, N., 2021. Effect of kinesio taping on low back pain during pregnancy: a systematic review and meta-analysis. *BMC Pregnancy and Childbirth*, 21, 1–11.

12